Managing Immunization in General Practice

Michael Ingram
General Practitioner
Hertfordshire

with a Foreword by
John Chisholm

RADCLIFFE MEDICAL PRESS
OXFORD AND NEW YORK

Radcliffe Medical Press Ltd
18 Marcham Road, Abingdon, Oxon OX14 1AA, UK

Radcliffe Medical Press, Inc.
141 Fifth Avenue, New York, NY 10010, USA

British Library Cataloguing in Publication Data

A catalogue record for this book is available from the British Library

ISBN 1 857751 55 8

Library of Congress Cataloging-in-Publication Data is available.

Typset by AMA Graphics Ltd., Preston
Printed and bound in Great Britain by Biddles Ltd., Guildford and King's Lynn

Contents

Acknowledgement

Thanks are due to Colin Gilligan and Robin Lowe, authors of *Marketing and General Practice*, Radcliffe Medical Press Ltd, 1995.

Foreword

Immunization is one of the few preventive interventions of undoubted and proven effectiveness. The US Preventive Services Task Force rightly assesses the evidence for a number of immunizations as being strongly supportable. Smallpox vaccination has entirely eradicated smallpox infection. Wild polio has been eradicated throughout the Western hemisphere. In the UK, dramatic reductions in childhood infectious diseases have been achieved through immunization, mostly now delivered by GPs and their primary health care teams. Recent examples of the contribution made in general practice to the achievement of public health policy objectives include the response made by family doctors to the target payment incentives of the 1990 GP contract and the early achievement of very high levels of uptake of *Haemophilus influenza* type b immunization, which have inevitably produced rapidly falling rates of infection.

GPs are thoroughly convinced of the public health arguments in favour of immunization and regard it as an integral part of their clinical practice. This book is designed to help them plan, provide, develop and monitor a comprehensive immunization service, not only for their NHS patients, but also, if they wish, on a private basis for travellers and for local companies. Good practice organization is the key to providing high quality clinical and preventive services, and this book is a notable and helpful contribution towards that good organization. It should help even the most efficient doctors to ensure that they are providing the best managed and most profitable immunization service they can—a service that should be welcomed by the patients it will benefit.

John Chisholm
February 1995

1

Introduction

Immunization is an activity that lies at the heart of general practice. This is particularly appropriate since it was a British rural practitioner who first discovered the effects of immunization against smallpox.

Immunization has become so familiar that it is generally taken for granted, yet administering a few drops of liquid or an injection offers invaluable protection to a vulnerable newborn child against diseases that were the constant fear of mothers in past centuries. At the other end of the spectrum, the elderly and the frail can be offered help in avoiding influenza and Pneumococcus infection; it is particularly poignant that many who are now receiving their annual 'flu jabs lived through the devastating influenza epidemic of 1919.

Immunization is developing constantly and bringing new solutions to existing problems. The last decade has seen important advances in the protection offered right across the age spectrum. Children are now immunized against *Haemophilus influenzae* type b, measles, mumps and rubella. A vaccine has been introduced to protect health service employees and others against the risk of hepatitis B, and more effective protection is now available against typhoid and hepatitis A. Massive resources are being channelled into developing further vaccines and into the search for the 'holy grail' of an effective vaccine against human immunodeficiency virus (HIV) infection, and there is the prospect that malaria may be at last brought under control through immunization.

However sophisticated the underlying research, vaccinating people is integral to general practice. Whilst academic researchers concentrate on developing new vaccines, in practice, when people want immunization for themselves, their children or elderly relatives, their first port of call is their GP. It is in general practice that they expect to get expert, independent advice about the need for immunization and where they will be given the vaccine by a familiar member of the practice team, with whom they are acquainted and feel at ease.

The central role of general practice in this field was well demonstrated in 1994. A mass immunization programme against measles and rubella was planned by the government, to be delivered through the school health service, with little, if any, participation by GPs. Yet, when parents learnt about these plans, it was to general practice that they turned for advice about whether or not their child should be immunized. Although this created an enormous amount of work for GPs, it was, nevertheless, flattering that parents should regard their GP as the best person to counsel them.

One other reason why immunization remains in general practice relates to the important matter of income. Immunization services are seen as being additional to the core of general medical services—the treatment of sick patients—and, therefore, attract various payments both within and outside the NHS. These provide an important source of income for GPs, and thus immunization is seen as an activity in which investment of time, resources and planning can bring increased financial reward. The fact that income is linked to providing immunization is a good example of how the profession can be encouraged to attain high standards of care if financial inducements are linked to a shared perception of the clinical value of the procedures being undertaken. This agreement, between those who determine health priorities and those who actually provide the care, is reassuring and something that is all too rarely seen in other areas of health care.

Given the high demand for immunization, the availability of safe and effective vaccines and the assurance of adequate income, it is clear why developing immunization services is not only desirable, but also vital to improving health care. Developing immunization services can be rewarding, both clinically and financially, and can be undertaken as fast and as far as practices wish.

Even within existing services, there is always scope to improve how they are being provided, through the elimination of wasteful practices, poor organization and loose financial management. Immunization is far too important to be left to reactive and ill thought-out systems. It requires a commitment from the practice team to ensure that the highest possible standards are pursued and achieved.

Within the practice, it is often the practice nurse who does most of the work with respect to immunization, although the service requires commitment from the whole practice team. Reception staff need to be familiar with the practice's policies and trained to give reliable and reassuring advice. Administrative staff need to handle and process records, claims and prescriptions, to ensure that the service is being delivered and that appropriate payments are claimed and received. The practice manager is likely to be in overall charge of the organization of the immunization service and should have a clear view of what the practice is seeking to achieve, how it is doing this and where efforts need to be concentrated. District nurses and health visitors can help by tackling problems arising from the need to immunize certain groups in the community and are a valuable resource to the practice. Likewise, the partners themselves need to be agreed on the purpose of the service and on the extent to which they are prepared to commit themselves to it and aware of the potential scope of the service being developed.

The management of an immunization service provides an ideal opportunity for the practice team to tackle a common task in a co-ordinated and thorough way, which can provide a template for co-operation, planning and management in other areas of the practice's work. Like many other tasks, the more effort that is put in, the greater the rewards in terms of job satisfaction and clinical and financial gains.

2

How to provide immunization services

Although good clinical skills are an essential prerequisite of high-quality general practice, they are not sufficient in themselves to ensure that patients receive a high standard of service. Recent changes within general practice have shown that GPs can no longer be regarded simply as clinicians; whether single handed or in partnership, fund holding or non-fund holding, all GPs have to recognize that basic organizational and managerial skills need to be applied to clinical practice. Even if GPs are unwilling to apply these themselves, someone else must be delegated to do so. There is much to gain by this. An efficiently run practice not only means fewer headaches for staff and doctors; equally importantly, it can ensure both increased income and increased professional satisfaction.

Immunization is a good example of this general principle. As part of a comprehensive immunization service, a practice should be providing:

- routine childhood immunization, which involves checking and rechecking whether or not targets are being reached, calling and recalling children and following up any defaulters

- travel immunization and travel-related services

- routine adult immunization

- immunization for those with a specific occupational or life-style risk, either within the practice population or as part of a company's occupational health service.

CLINICS

A key decision that has to be taken is whether or not to base the immunization service in clinics, each being run for a specific immunization programme.

Advantages

▓ Each clinic can cover a specific task (unlike most of general practice, where patient needs vary from one consultation to the next).

▓ Any paperwork can be batched and more efficiently processed.

▓ Protocols can be introduced more easily.

▓ Additional needs can be met and information offered; for example, a health visitor can run an advice session as part of a baby vaccination clinic, or travel kits can be sold to private patients at a travel clinic.

▓ Multidose vials can save costs (though may have a short life span).

▓ Clinics can be run at times that particularly suit certain patients, for example travel clinics in evenings and on Saturday mornings.

▓ Large numbers of immunizations can be administered quickly, as may be required in an influenza programme.

Disadvantages

▓ Because many patients have busy lives, they find it difficult to attend clinics run on specific days and at fixed times; any difficulty in attending may be compounded by their reluctance to be immunized.

▓ Immunizations that are given infrequently cannot be grouped together into a clinic; for example, it would be difficult to organize a regular occupational health immunization clinic convenient to patients.

▒ Receptionists may be tempted to pressurize patients to use a clinic even if it is inconvenient to them; this can increase the level of non-attendance.

▒ Some nurses (and doctors) find it boringly repetitive to have a continuous flow of patients attending for the same reason.

OPPORTUNISTIC IMMUNIZATION

A particularly effective way of providing an immunization service is to make it an integral part of the practice's normal routine. One area in which this approach can easily be adopted is during the routine checks and clinics already operating. There are several such opportunities for offering immunization (Table 2.1). Information given by patients attending these clinics can reveal clinical conditions for which immunization may be required. Practice nurses running these clinics should be encouraged to recognize the need for these immunizations

Table 2.1:   Arcas for opportunistic immunization in general practice

New patient check	Check on immunization status and offer tetanus booster and polio, and also hepatitis B if relevant to occupation
Practice nurse clinic	Tetanus if wound is dressed or treated
Children's clinic	Polio course to unimmunized parents if child is having polio course
Chronic disease	Pneumococcus and influenza immunizations can be targeted at patients attending asthma and diabetes clinics
Over-75 patient check	Opportunity for tetanus course or booster and influenza or Pneumococcus vaccine
Waiting room area	Poster campaign; familiarity of reception staff with basic information about immunizations

and to ensure that they are provided immediately, thereby avoiding having to recall the patient for a second visit.

There is also scope for reception staff to recognize opportunities for immunization; there are times when patients mention something to the receptionist that points to a need for immunization, for example reference to a forthcoming holiday, the acquisition of a pet (more relevant to a tetanus booster than rabies!) or looking after a newly born grandchild. It is reasonable to encourage reception staff to be aware of these opportunities and advise patients to discuss their immunization requirements with the practice nurse.

Most opportunistic immunization arises from the normal doctor–patient consultation. The uptake of vaccines, such as those against influenza, tetanus, polio and Pneumococcus, can be greatly increased if the doctor recommends them. However, if opportunistic immunization is to be integrated successfully into routine surgery consultations, the following points should be addressed.

▧ The GP must keep immunization in mind, even though patients are consulting on a widely varying range of conditions.

▧ Offering immunizations during routine consultations lengthens them. Deciding whether a vaccination is needed, discussing it with the patient, explaining its side-effects and finally administering the vaccine can all add substantially to the length of a consultation (even though the practice nurse may carry out the administration). There is the further risk that some patients are drawn into a complex discussion of the pros and cons of being immunized.

▧ Because it is necessary to make a rapid decision on whether or not a particular immunization is appropriate, the GP must have ready access to authoritative advice.

▧ Ideally, vaccines should be stored in a refrigerator in each consulting room, although this can create difficulties with stock control. Alternatively, the reception staff can set aside the small number of doses likely to be used during a normal surgery in a cool box. (Again, these problems are circumvented if the patient is referred to the practice nurse for the vaccine to be administered.).

▧ Many GPs are less thorough than are their practice staff when dealing with the paperwork—there must be a foolproof system that ensures that claim forms are completed and prescriptions issued.

APPOINTMENT SYSTEMS FOR IMMUNIZATIONS

The most common way of providing immunizations is for patients to consult the practice nurse; the length of each consultation must ensure that there is enough time to give any clinical advice and to assess any other immunization needs.

Childhood immunization

Childhood immunizations are important both clinically and financially. The contribution made by population immunization to eradicating and reducing the incidence of common infectious diseases is well documented. The incidence of measles has been dramatically reduced following the introduction of vaccines, a trend that was temporarily reversed following the vaccine scare of the mid-1970s. More recently, the fall in childhood infections caused by *Haemophilus influenzae* following the introduction of Hib vaccine has again demonstrated the powerful effects of childhood immunization.

The target payments associated with both the primary course of immunizations and pre-school boosters form a significant proportion of total practice income, particularly if the higher level payments are achieved. Because these payments are devised to reward good clinical practice, both clinical and financial grounds can be used to justify putting considerable effort into achieving these targets.

A practice should aim to immunize all of its child patients, but the prospect of achieving this objective depends on how the service is run and on the population it serves.

High deprivation areas can present major problems; patient turnover makes record-keeping difficult, and some parents may lack the motivation and organization to attend with their children when requested. Sadly, poverty and overcrowding make these children more vulnerable to the diseases against which immunization is being offered. In these areas, practices have to devote far greater resources to their childhood immunization service.

Patients should be offered as many opportunities as are practicable for their children to receive the required immunizations.

▨ Clinics should be held at regular times on fixed days, so that parents know when to come.

▓ Parents should not be discouraged from dropping in opportunistically if necessary.

▓ Clinic times should be convenient to parents; during mid-mornings siblings may be at nursery, play group or school and mothers may, therefore, find it easier to attend.

▓ Opportunistic immunization should be offered whenever an unimmunized child attends surgery, even if he or she is merely accompanying a parent.

▓ Immunization clinics should be linked to health visitor consultations.

▓ An interpreter or link worker should be available where there is a significant number of ethnic minority patients.

Central administration and call and recall systems can ease a practice's administrative tasks. Health authority computer-based lists can be produced for each clinic, and each child can be invited to attend. However, errors do occur, and the clinic list should be checked carefully for these. Staff may notice wrong names or addresses that will prevent letters being delivered and may know of families who are likely not to attend and need to be reminded by telephone or even require a home visit.

Most practices should have their own recall system for childhood immunizations. Nevertheless, it is advisable to review progress with the practice's health visitors to compare health authority and practice data and identify those children who have not been immunized. Computerization has meant that there is easier access to data, and most software contains the necessary search facilities.

By running these checks, a practice can estimate whether or not it is likely to meet its immunization targets each quarter and identify any defaulting children. This applies to both primary immunizations and pre-school boosters.

MEETING TARGETS

In financial terms, it is vital for a practice to meet its childhood immunization targets; this is why good administrative and call and recall systems are so important. There are several ways in which targets can be achieved.

▓ Identifying the target population. The children in the patient population base for the targets should be listed. By scrutinizing the list of names, those families that are most likely to default can be identified. In addition, some children may have been wrongly included due to an incorrect date of birth, or families who have moved away may have failed to register elsewhere. There are particular problems in areas with a high patient turnover, because the health authority and practice lists may differ considerably. An additional problem can occur among ethnic minorities, where similar names, naming conventions and parents' command of the English language all lead to health authorities misidentifying children on the practice list.

▓ Checking that the immunizations have been given. This can often be done by a computer search. Whichever method is used, the practice must ensure that it has managed to complete enough immunization courses to meet its targets. Sometimes the central child health records resolve any doubts over which doses of which vaccine have been given.

▓ Creating a 'hit list' of all those children who have not completed their immunization course and making a determined effort to vaccinate them.

▓ Making sure that the parent or guardian of every child has actually been contacted with an offer of immunization.

▓ Making sure that immunization has been properly offered before assuming that it has been refused. The doctor should talk to the parent or guardian directly, either at the surgery or by telephone, and the doctor or health visitor should visit if necessary to combat any anxieties about immunization. The practice may wish to seek advice from a community paediatrician if there are complex issues that the parents wish to raise.

▓ Telephoning parents after any failure to attend, to discuss the reason and to arrange a further appointment.

▓ Offering domiciliary visits, either by the practice nurse, health visitor or GP if all other avenues have been explored. This effective (but labour intensive) approach may be essential if a practice is close to reaching its targets and other efforts to achieve compliance have failed.

▨ Monitoring progress via a regular manual or computer search.

A practice should ensure that it does everything possible within its time and staffing constraints to meet its targets. Health visitors can have a crucial role in chasing up defaulters and explaining the importance of immunization. In addition, there may be local ethnic link workers who can help with language difficulties. There may, however, be some practices in which all these efforts are simply not cost-effective, because they do not have a realistic prospect of ever reaching the higher target levels. Such practices may reluctantly decide to give up bothering to chase defaulters. It is to be hoped that such decisions are comparatively rare.

When everything has been tried, there may be some families who persist in refusing immunization for their children. Parents who hold these views can threaten the achievement of target payments. Some practices believe that they are justified in removing these families from their lists. Such action, however, is ill advised. The GMC advises that it is unacceptable to discriminate against patients because of their perceived economic worth. Nonetheless, doctors have a right to remove patients from their lists when they perceive that the doctor–patient relationship has irretrievably broken down.

Paperwork

One advantage of childhood immunization is that it involves less bureaucracy than that associated with item of service fees for immunization. However, because of the 'all or nothing' way in which the target system works, any administrative errors can be very costly. The following procedures should ensure that targets are not missed because of an omission.

▨ Ensuring that child health immunization sheets are completed when the injections are given.

▨ Keeping copies of all sheets in case of any dispute over targets.

▨ Ensuring that completed sheets are sent to the health authority by courier or recorded delivery post.

▓ Entering immunizations on to the practice's computer system, using a member of staff who has specific responsibility for this task; he or she should also check that the immunizations have been recorded in the patients' notes.

GENERAL IMMUNIZATION

Other immunizations are difficult to organize into clinics because they are given infrequently, often when suggested by a doctor or nurse rather than because the patient asks for them.

The best way of offering adult immunizations within general practice is to integrate them into routine surgeries and clinics; for example, opportunistic immunization can be offered during normal consultations. This is particularly appropriate for routine influenza immunizations, because patients with chronic diseases tend to consult more frequently and can be easily approached during consultations. This same principle can be applied to tetanus immunizations, which can also be offered opportunistically during consultations, for example as a spring offensive as patients are emerging into their gardens!

An exception to this approach is the large scale influenza immunization campaign. A clearly delineated patient population should be offered regular annual immunization at a specific time of year. Clinics should be used for this because many patients who need this vaccine have retired from work and can attend during the day and because batch processing of prescriptions and clinical entries is more efficient. There is also scope for providing Pneumococcus vaccine at influenza clinics, because there is a substantial overlap between the populations at risk of these two diseases.

TRAVEL IMMUNIZATION

Travel immunization is an expanding area of general practice, and it should be provided as a comprehensive service at times that are convenient to patients. Some practices have concentrated on providing travel clinics, whilst others have simply included travel immunizations in their practice nurse services.

Good organization is essential. If a practice is considering running a travel immunization service, it needs to base its decision on an objective assessment of several key issues. Key questions include the following.

▓ What are the aims of the proposed travel immunization service?

— How can those patients travelling overseas be identified and their risks assessed?

— How can ill health be prevented while abroad, through prophylactic immunization?

▓ How should the new service be run?

— Should it be based around separate clinics?

— What is the likely level of demand for it?

— How long should individual appointments be?

— When should appointments be offered?

— Should weekend or evening sessions be organized?

▓ What information sources should be used?

— Should reference books, telephone lines or on-line databases be employed?

▓ What should be the scale of fees charged?

▓ Will the practice's current equipment and facilities be sufficient?

▓ What training is required for staff, in particular practice nurses?

It helps to have a protocol setting out the procedures to be undertaken; this involves deciding:

▓ what use should be made of a questionnaire for obtaining information about patients prior to the consultation

▓ what reference sources should be used

▓ what advice should be provided during the appointment

▓ what the practice's policies on prescribing and providing malaria prophylaxis should be

- which contraindications and side-effects of immunizations should be explained to patients

- how travel clinic consultations should be recorded in patients' notes

- what equipment or kits should be recommended

- when patients should be referred by a practice nurse to a doctor.

The more comprehensive the protocol, the more protection it gives to practice staff, particularly practice nurses, who usually undertake most of this work.

The actual process of preparing and introducing a protocol should ensure that everyone involved in the travel immunization service has the opportunity to express views on how it should run.

Yellow fever immunization

This can only be given at designated official yellow fever immunization centres; any practice wishing to be authorized should apply to the Department of Health[1]. The DoH looks for certain minimum standards that ensure the vaccine is stored safely and administered correctly; applicants also have to show that they can administer the clinic efficiently. Immunization against yellow fever is not an NHS service. Because a practice recognized as a yellow fever centre is not con-strained by its NHS terms of service, it can:

- charge patients, including its NHS patients, for the service

- treat patients from other practices that are not yellow fever centres

- set charges at whatever level it chooses

- separate charges for administering the vaccination from those for issuing the certificate.

---

[1]International Relations Unit, Department of Health, Room 554, Richmond House, 79 Whitehall, London SW1A 2NS.
In Scotland: Scottish Home and Health Department, St Andrew's House, Regent Road, Edinburgh EH1 3DG.

The yellow fever vaccine, although purchased by the practice, is specifically excluded from reimbursement under the personal administration scheme, so patients' fees must cover its cost.

During the last few years, more practices have become yellow fever centres; some areas are so well provided for that price competition has set in. Therefore, practice income from yellow fever centre immunization has declined in relative terms and it is becoming a less attractive source of income.

Minimum standards for a yellow fever centre include the following.

▓ Storage and administration of vaccine should comply with the requirements set out in *Immunization Against Infectious Disease* (The Green Book)[2].

▓ Vaccines must be approved by the WHO.

▓ An authorized GP must be in charge (although vaccination can be delegated to a practice nurse).

▓ The international certificate against yellow fever must be signed by an authorized doctor.

▓ Certificates must comply with the international health regulations model.

▓ Paper records of all immunizations must be kept.

▓ The practice must have an official stamp approved by the Department of Health.

▓ The Department of Health must be told of any changes and be able to inspect the centre at any time.

CALL AND RECALL

Experience shows that some patients seem to be unable to comply with instructions on the frequency or duration of a course of treatment, to attend for review of a chronic condition or even to keep an appointment they made that same day! Hence, effective call and recall systems are needed.

---

[2]*Immunization Against Infectious Disease*, HMSO, London.

Call systems

These ask patients to attend for a procedure to be initiated, for example childhood immunization in which the initiative Is taken by a health authority. Practices may wish to use their own call systems. All new notes should be reviewed, so that patients who appear not to have undergone a tetanus or polio immunization course can be called. Similarly, evidence of occupational or life-style risk factors could justify a call for hepatitis B immunization.

A disadvantage is that 'calls' do not work if there is no perceived need. Although parents will respond to a call for their child to be vaccinated, they may ignore a letter asking them to attend for a tetanus booster or hepatitis B course. Practices that call patients routinely should monitor the response rate, assessing the need for the vaccine among those who do not respond and estimating whether or not any revenue subsequently earned covers the administrative and postage costs of the call system.

Recall systems

Many patients fail to attend for subsequent doses of an immunization course or forget that a booster dose is due. This often occurs if several courses are being provided or if there is a long gap between doses, as, for example, with hepatitis B immunizations. Also, if travel vaccines are being given, patients often associate these with the holiday itself, and, as its memory fades, they forget that their immunization course has not been completed.

An efficient recall system ensures that:

▧ the patient benefits from the protection of a completed immunization course

▧ the patient does not mistakenly assume that the immunization is complete

▧ the practice has discharged its duty of care to the patient

▧ the practice reaps maximum income for its efforts, particularly since booster doses usually attract the higher fee.

Recall systems are as good as the data they use. Many practices prefer a paper-based system, which may seem easier to understand to some GPs than a computerized system. However, the advantages of computerized recall and dispatch of letters are considerable in ease of use and time saved.

Paper-based recall

A card index is all that is needed; patients' details, together with the stages reached in the immunization courses are recorded and the cards should be filed according to the date the next dose is due. At the end of the week, those patients who have missed their follow-up appointments are contacted by letter or telephone. Telephone contact (particularly if it is made by the GP!) is often more effective and has the additional advantage of allowing an appointment to be arranged immediately.

Attempts at recall should be noted in the patient's records in case of any subsequent complaint from the patient.

Computerized recall

Most GP computer software includes recall systems; if a recall option is not available, the software supplier should be asked to provide one. All data should be entered on the computer by the person giving the immunization or by a designated computer operator; the latter option avoids the somewhat sloppy and idiosyncratic habits of some doctors!

Whether it is computerized or paper based, any recall system benefits from a clearly defined procedure. This should include:

- putting one person (with a deputy) in charge of the system

- deciding how often recalls are sent or made by telephone

- deciding how many defaults are tolerable and what further action, if any, should be taken.

RECORD-KEEPING

If GPs were no longer paid item of service fees for the immunizations, but were instead paid according to how many patients claimed that they did not know how many vaccinations they had had or how long ago they had had them, GPs' income could be greatly enhanced! This point is made to stress the importance of recording immunizations accurately and clearly. Two recording systems should be used: one in the practice, on the patient's NHS notes and computer record, and the other on a record card retained by the patient. The NHS notes should contain a separate card that records immunizations and allows easy reference to the patient's vaccination status. Essential features include:

▓ recording the date of immunization and the type and batch of vaccine

▓ the inclusion of new vaccines as they become available

▓ simplicity and legibility

▓ a size of card that fits neatly into an NHS Lloyd George envelope.

An example of a card used in the author's practice is illustrated in Figure 2.1.

Patient-held records vary. Some are supplied by pharmaceutical companies. Unfortunately, there is no UK equivalent of the French carnet, which provides a full immunization history and seems to be diligently guarded by French citizens. However, most patients care for records entrusted to them, as many a dog-eared tetanus vaccination card extracted from a wallet will testify. Durability and a credit card size are laudable characteristics of any patient card.

There are medicolegal implications of record keeping. Failure to record doses and batch numbers makes it difficult to defend any legal action arising from an adverse reaction or a claim that there was an error in the type or dose of vaccine administered. These important considerations have become more relevant, as is evident from the recent withdrawal of one of a variety of MMR vaccines because of potential side-effects and from the increasing litigation resulting from brain damage allegedly caused by the pertussis vaccine. Batch numbers are essential in ensuring that any claim can be directed towards the supplier rather than the practice.

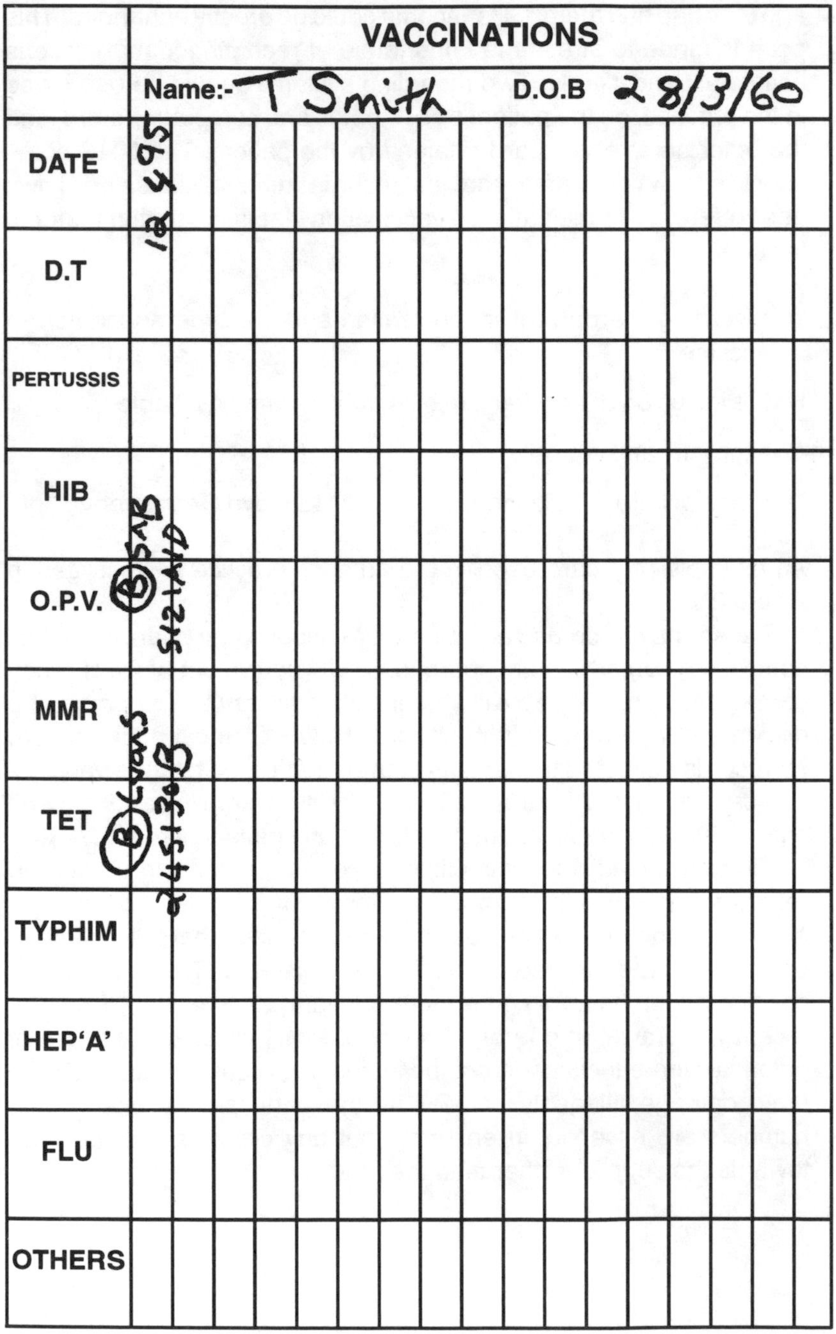

VACCINATIONS																	
	Name:- T Smith					D.O.B 28/3/60											
DATE	18 495 81																
D.T																	
PERTUSSIS																	
HIB																	
O.P.V.	⑧5x15 5121 AHD																
MMR																	
TET	⑧ Evans 24513068																
TYPHIM																	
HEP'A'																	
FLU																	
OTHERS																	

Figure 2.1: A general practice vaccination record card.

3

The role of the practice team

Members of the practice team, particularly practice nurses who often do most of the work, play a crucial role in providing immunization services.

THE PRACTICE NURSE

Practice nurses are particularly well suited to running the immunization service because:

- they are trained to comply with the procedures and protocols of an immunization service

- they are efficient at tasks that lie within their specialty

- patients sometimes see them as more caring and sympathetic than doctors, and as having more time to listen

- they deal efficiently with paperwork, including call and recall systems and forms

- a proportion of their salary is usually directly reimbursed by the health authority or health board

▓ they can act as a 'scapegoat' for childhood immunization: because the child does not associate a doctor with the injection, future consultations with the child are made somewhat easier

▓ their profession has traditionally been heavily involved in this type of work.

Developing protocols

Practice nurses have an important role in developing an immunization service, whether it is focused on travel, adult or childhood risks, and should be closely involved in any review of a practice's immunization policy. Because they actually carry out the immunizing, they are best able to identify problems in existing arrangements and to assess how patients will react to any change.

Opportunistic immunization

In their day-to-day work, practice nurses treat many people who could benefit from immunization: the elderly, the chronically sick and patients attending the practice's diabetic and asthma clinics. They are, therefore, ideally placed to initiate immunization. Patients respect the practice nurse's advice when encouraged to protect themselves against diseases such as tetanus, polio, hepatitis B and influenza.

Developing the service

Practice nurses should be encouraged to suggest how the service might be improved. The development of new vaccines will itself lead to change: for example, the recent introduction of low-dose combined diphtheria and tetanus vaccine for school leavers, and of acellular pertussis and diphtheria vaccines for travellers, has increased the demand for immunizations. Practice nurses should be encouraged to monitor new developments in immunization, with a view to introducing these to the practice. Of course, doctors themselves cannot entirely devolve to their nurses responsibility for the clinical care of patients; they should also keep abreast of new developments.

Telephone advice

Practice nurses can give telephone advice on immunization; for example, they can tell patients who need travel immunizations when they should come to the surgery and what the immunizations involve and can discuss with anxious parents their children's vaccinations. In general, patients should be encouraged to recognize nurses' expertise, because this enables them to play a much larger role in the practice and, in particular, to assist the GPs when there is sudden widespread anxiety among patients, as is sometimes caused by the withdrawal of a vaccine or the introduction of a government-initiated immunization programme, such as the 1994 measles/rubella campaign.

The practice nurse's role

Practice nurses should:

- know the limits of their capabilities, ensuring that they turn to authoritative reference sources or seek advice from the GPs if they are in doubt

- contribute fully to developing and implementing practice protocols and participate in any review of them

- be responsible for their own actions, on the understanding that the employing GPs are ultimately liable for any acts or omissions

- ensure they maintain their skills and knowledge through continuing education

- advise and assist other practice team members as and when required

- maintain the stock of vaccines and help to ensure that these are bought at the most economic price, subject to any preferences expressed by the GPs.

Practice nurses welcome freedom from the hierarchical constraints of hospital and community nursing services and in response to this greatly increased autonomy, they are usually willing to accept increased responsibility for organizing their own day-to-day professional work.

On the other hand, GP employers of practice nurses should:

■ provide training in immunization, including refresher courses

■ accept ultimate responsibility for any acts or omissions

■ provide sufficient medical support, by making themselves available to give advice and assistance

■ address any anxieties about shortcomings or deficiencies in the immunization service

■ ensure that fees charged to patients are both consistent and reasonable.

Practice nurses cannot prescribe immunizations, so there must be a prescribing procedure that enables nurses to immunize patients as and when required. This may be based on various arrangements, such as individual prescribing, individual authorization or, perhaps most efficiently, a group protocol (see Chapter 8 for an explanation of how this can operate).

There are many opportunities for practice nurse training in immunization; details can be obtained from the Royal College of Nursing (RCN) or the Central Council for Nursing, Midwifery and Health Visiting.

There should also be training in post, as the learning process can be far more effective if reinforced in the day-to-day work of the practice.

Stock control

Practice nurses should be responsible for ordering and maintaining the stock of vaccines. This task requires them to ensure that sufficient supplies are available and that vaccines are properly stored and not used beyond their expiry date. Because vaccines must be stored below room temperature (and within a specified temperature range), nurses should follow a storage protocol to ensure that vaccines are not damaged by inadequate temperature control. This protocol can also be used to tell other staff how to handle stock. As part of the protocol, refrigeration equipment should be checked regularly to ensure that it is working correctly, for example by recording the minimum/maximum thermometer readings of each refrigerator in a log book.

RECEPTION STAFF

Reception staff are the front line, being the first point of contact for patients enquiring about immunization, booking appointments and attending clinics; reception staff have a vital role in the service. Patients judge a practice by their first impressions and its external appearance. This does not apply just to the immunization service: the practice should ensure that all patients are dealt with promptly, efficiently and courteously.

Because reception staff help to implement immunization procedures, they should be encouraged to contribute to developing these, by expressing views on:

▓ the length of individual appointments for immunization

▓ the frequency and timing of clinics, with a view to avoiding any overload at peak times

▓ the procedures for answering telephone enquiries

▓ the policy for repeat bookings, follow-up and missed appointments.

Advice to patients from reception staff

The practice has to decide who should advise patients, whether face to face or by telephone. Reception staff should be trained to give basic advice (e.g. by referring to an immunization chart and telling patients which immunizations are recommended and which are obligatory). Involving reception staff in this work can ensure that the practice nurses' skills and time are deployed more effectively.

Training of reception staff should ensure that they:

▓ understand the importance attached to immunization: any task is much more rewarding if its purpose is understood

▓ appreciate the contribution of immunization in preventing disease, especially for children and those adults whose travel, life-style or occupation carries special risks

▓ understand the contribution that immunization makes to practice income; the essential principles of the target schemes should be explained, together with the importance of travel immunizations as a source of income

▓ realize that subsequent doses in a course and booster doses are as important as are original doses, and should be given at the time prescribed in the protocol

▓ know how to answer enquiries by referring to up-to-date information on recommended immunization and malaria prophylaxis. (This may be obtained from the immunization tables published in the weekly GP papers)

▓ are capable of explaining the difference between obligatory and recommended immunizations. (Reception staff should tell patients the importance of complying with the recommended prophylaxis and should know when to seek help from a practice nurse or GP if further clarification or persuasion is required)

▓ know when to seek advice from or refer to a practice nurse or doctor

▓ understand the basic immunization protocols, so that appointments and follow-ups are correctly booked. (They should also ensure that mothers are aware of the importance of a return visit for their children's next injection)

▓ understand and follow an agreed protocol that specifies their duties and responsibilities

▓ be aware of the need for travel advice and the need to raise the subject with patients whenever an appropriate opportunity occurs, for example:

— if a repeat prescription is requested early or for an increased volume of drugs because the patient is going on holiday

— when a patient asks for a passport form to be countersigned

— when a patient asks for a health report for travel, for kibbutz work or for a 'freedom from infection' certificate.

THE PRACTICE MANAGER

An immunization service inevitably increases the practice's administrative work, and the practice manager has considerable influence over how this is handled. Because the practice manager's wholehearted co-operation is vital, he or she should be closely involved in organizing the service and should play a key part in any discussions about how it might be changed. His or her responsibilities include:

▓ planning clinic sessions, allocating rooms and ensuring that staff and equipment are available

▓ setting up administrative systems for making appointments, giving telephone advice, processing claim forms, checking that forms are completed and dispatched and ensuring that all payments are promptly received

▓ dealing with staffing matters.

Obviously, the practice manager delegates many tasks to other staff, but he or she should ultimately be responsible for the overall management of the immunization service.

HEALTH VISITORS

Health visitors have a statutory duty to visit children under five years of age, and their involvement in the practice's immunization service should be concentrated upon childhood immunizations. Because they are employed by a health authority or NHS community trust and not by the practice, they provide a valued additional source of help in managing immunization.

Health visitors should be asked to assist with problems in the area of childhood immunization, especially if families are either failing to attend or refusing to allow their children to be vaccinated. Health visitors may be willing to visit parents at home to discuss these problems and to help with tracing families who have moved.

The health visitor's work could be extended to include immunizing patients in their own homes if there is no other feasible alternative. The extent of their responsibilities and functions varies according to the area in which they work; in high-deprivation areas, they may be more involved in local practices' childhood immunization campaigns.

Health visitors may also be willing to become involved in clinics. Immunization compliance can be greatly improved if childhood vaccines are given alongside other child health services in 'one-stop' clinics. Health visitors can run baby weighing and checking clinics alongside the practice's immunization clinics, making both services more accessible to mothers.

All health visitors are familiar with the usual childhood immunizations; however, those working in socially deprived areas or areas with significant ethnic minority populations should be familiar with additional prophylactic injections. For example, in such areas, BCG vaccination is particularly important because of the increased incidence of tuberculosis, owing to poverty and poor living conditions. The health visitor should follow up any defaulters. Another example is immunization against hepatitis B; this has recently been introduced on a routine basis for children of certain ethnic groups that carry an above-average risk of the virus. This immunization programme is likely to be expanded, because the World Health Organization (WHO) has decreed that countries with lower carrier rates, such as the UK, should introduce routine immunization by 1997. When this happens, health visitors will need to help with the programme in the same way that they have done so effectively with the measles, mumps and rubella (MMR) and *Haemophilus influenzae* type b (Hib) programmes.

4

Financial issues

For most GPs, the NHS is their major source of income for immunization work. Any growth in income from this source depends not only on expanding their immunization service, but also on administrative systems that ensure that all payments due are being claimed.

Although the GPs' pay system does not actually restrict individual NHS income, if all GPs maximized their earnings from a particular activity, such as immunization work, the Review Body would seek to counteract this. The Pay Review Body tries to ensure that average GP earnings in general practices are maintained at a given level; thus, if there is an increase in earnings across the profession as a whole in excess of the Pay Review Body's recommended figure; fees and allowances are subsequently adjusted to contain the increase and claw back any excess. In theory, if all doctors doubled their item of service income from immunization, it could result in halving of the fees paid for this work! The only current exception, as described below, is the treatment of higher target premiums.

There are three main sources of NHS income.

▓ Target payments are bonus payments for achieving targets in immunization coverage, in both primary courses and pre-school boosters. The amount payable depends on the number of children vaccinated and who does the work.

▓ Item of service payments are earned for certain other immunizations, in accordance with public policy. The fee scale provides for two levels of fee, depending on whether the immunization is part of a basic course, a completing dose or a booster.

▓ Payments for personal administration of immunizations are only available to GP practices in England and Wales.

TARGET PAYMENTS

Target payments are made for reaching target levels of immunization coverage in:

▓ the primary immunization course, consisting of diphtheria, tetanus and pertussis (the triple vaccine), polio, Hib and MMR vaccines

▓ the pre-school booster, consisting of diphtheria, tetanus and polio vaccines.

The present schedule of primary immunization is shown in Table 4.1.
    Any practice seeking to increase its earnings from immunization must look to its target payments and understand how the scheme works.

Table 4.1:   Current schedule of primary immunization

	Age (months)		
Diphtheria, tetanus and pertussis (triple)	2	3	4
Polio	2	3	4
Hib	2	3	4
MMR	12–18		

Primary immunizations: how the payment system works

▓ Payments are only made if targets are achieved.

▓ There is a higher fee for the 90% target and a lower one for the 70% target.

▨ Every injection completing the primary immunization course — namely the third doses of pertussis, diphtheria, tetanus, polio and Hib, and the one vaccination of MMR — counts towards the calculation of targets. As long as the first two doses have been given, it is financially irrelevant where or by whom they were administered.

▨ The target population will include all children on the practice list who are two years old on the first day of the quarter.

▨ The calculation is made as shown in Table 4.2.

▨ The payment is proportioned to the work carried out in general medical services. If there are 22 children aged two years on a doctor's list, the 90% target has been reached by their being immunized, and the immunizations were entirely administered in general practice (either in the current or a previous practice), the fee paid will be the higher payment quoted in the Red Book. If a 70% target is reached under the same conditions, the lower payment, which is one-third of the value of the higher payment is received.

▨ If there are more than 22 children on the practice list, the target payment is proportionately higher. However, immunizations given outside general practice will lead to a reduced payment (Table 4.2).

Although in this case the calculations are similar, they are much simpler, because they are based on the number of children who have had their pre-school booster of diphtheria, tetanus and polio. The target population is the number of five-year-olds on the practice list at the start of each quarter. Again, achievement of the 90% target earns a bonus payment three times that paid for reaching the 70% target.

It is important to remember that the total earnings of GPs as a whole are limited to the 'pool' of income based on the Review Body award. Because GPs' target net remuneration only includes the lower target payments, and because the difference between the higher and lower targets (the higher target premium payment) is not included in average net remuneration, the profession as a whole earns new money from the higher target fees; as more GPs meet these higher targets, the total earnings of the profession will increase.

Table 4.2:   Target payments

Four doctor practice with 100 two-year-olds

Total number of 2 year olds in practice on 1 September   = 100
Maximum possible number of completing immunizations
   possible 100 × 4 (100 children each having a completing   = 400
   dose of DT and polio, pertussis, Hib and MMR)
so 90% target requires 360 completing doses
or 70% target requires 280 completing doses

If the total number of completing immunizations actually achieved = 369
    92 had DT and polio
    86 had pertussis   All were administered in general practice
    95 had Hib
    96 had MMR
Therefore, 90% target has been reached

90 % target reached so should get £2145/doctor/year = £2145 per quarter

But 25 children per doctor, not 22
so $\dfrac{25}{22} \times £2145 = £2437.50$

However only 90 can count in each group so payment has to be reduced by
calculating 90 + 86 + 90 + 90 = 356
£2437.50 is reduced by $\dfrac{356}{360} \times £2437.50 = £2410.42$

The practice will receive £2410.42 if all jabs were given in general practice

However, if 10 doses of each group are given in a clinic:
    82 had DT and polio in general practice
    78 had pertussis in general practice
    85 had Hib in general practice
    86 had MMR in general practice
Total in general practice is 331

90% target needs 360 in all so payment by proportion $\dfrac{331}{360} = 0.919$

Thus the practice will actually receive £2410.42 × 0.919 = £2215.18

OTHER INCOME FROM CHILDHOOD IMMUNIZATION

There is no other source of income from childhood immunizations as such, apart from the target payment scheme. Practices can no longer purchase the vaccine directly, because it is now supplied centrally. However, some indirect sources of income are outlined below.

Polio

The risk of other persons contracting polio should be seriously assessed. The oral polio vaccine virus passes through the child's gut, and occasionally an adult contracts polio from contact with a baby's faeces when changing a nappy. It is therefore important to check that both parents and anyone else in contact with a nappy (e.g. grand-parents, other relatives, nannies and au pairs) have had a full course of polio immunization. If not, they should be immunized, and an item of service fee should be claimed.

Tetanus

If someone has not had a primary polio course, it is probable that he or she had also missed a tetanus injection and therefore requires a primary tetanus course, for which item of service fees and payments for the personal administration of the vaccine can be claimed.

Registration and child health surveillance

When a child patient is immunized, here is an ideal opportunity to confirm that no other potential source of income is being overlooked. Checks should be carried out to ensure that:

- the child is actually registered with the practice and that form FP58 has been received. If the child is not registered, target payments, as well as capitation fees, may be lost

- the child health surveillance claim form has been signed.

ITEM OF SERVICE FEES

Rules governing these fees are in paragraph 27 of the Red Book; they specify which patients, which immunizations and which doses can be claimed for.

Which patients?

To claim an immunization fee, the patient must be:

■ on the doctor's own list

or

■ on a partner's list

or

■ eligible for treatment as a temporary resident

or

■ in the practice area for not more than 24 hours.

These rules allow some flexibility and scope for running an immunization service for those people who might otherwise not have access to one; for example, an inner city practice could run a vaccination clinic for commuters who work nearby and be paid for this work on the same basis as if they were treating their own registered patients.

It also means that a doctor can offer an immunization service to some patients of other practices. However, before doing so, the doctor should ensure that this will not be viewed with hostility by neighbouring practices. Any immunizations provided when working as an employee of a local health authority, or as a school medical officer, are not eligible for item of service fees (even if the doctor is treating his or her own patients).

There are some occupational groups whose work carries special risks for whom an immunization fee can be claimed; these include:

■ health workers, for whom fees for diphtheria and polio boosters at regular intervals can be claimed

▓ workers in woollen mills, tanneries and glue and bonemeal facto-
ries, who may need anthrax immunization if handling imported raw
materials

▓ those working with imported live mammals or inspecting quaran-
tine quarters, who need rabies immunization.

Eligible immunizations

The Red Book lists those immunizations for which a health authority
or the Health Board pays an item of service fee. The fee is at two
levels, referred to as 'A' and 'B'. The immunizations for which these
fees are paid are shown in Table 4.3.

The list in the Red Book reads like a vestige from a bygone era,
having little relevance to current clinical practice and taking little or no
account of new developments in immunization. For example, a fee

Table 4.3:   'A' and 'B' fee immunizations

Fee 'A'	Fee 'B'
First typhoid	Typhoid booster (include Typhim Vi)
All cholera	Immunoglobulin
Polio 1 and 2	Polio 3 and booster
Tetanus 1 and 2	Tetanus 3 and booster
Diphtheria 1 and 2	Diptheria 3 and booster
	MMR (unimmunized children aged 6 to 15)
	Measles (unimmunized children aged 6 to 15)
	Rubella
	Active hepatitis A
Anthrax 1, 2 and 3	Anthrax 4 and booster
Typhoid 1 and 2	Typhoid booster
Rabies 1	Rabies 2 and booster
Cholera	

can still be claimed for smallpox immunization, even though the WHO has declared that the disease has been eradicated and it is not even possible to obtain the vaccine! Cholera vaccination still attracts a fee, even though the WHO no longer endorses immunization because it lacks efficacy.

On the other hand, hepatitis B is not even mentioned in the Red Book. This represents a serious deficiency, because there are important public health issues at stake. The WHO is pressing for this vaccine to be included in routine childhood immunization programmes in the UK by 1997. Furthermore, even when the government's guidelines require immunization, no fee is payable.

Other anomalies relate to geographical areas; for example, only the northern countries of Europe are ineligible when claiming a fee for hepatitis A and typhoid immunizations; thus a fee is paid for immunizing someone against hepatitis A and typhoid who is travelling to Switzerland, a country that is hardly renowned for its insanitary conditions!

Further complications arise from health authorities and health boards' different interpretations of the Red Book, as shown in the examples below.

■ The new Vi polysaccharide antigen typhoid vaccine is a single dose, and, although it is not specifically referred to in the Red Book, most health authorities interpret this as being eligible for the higher fee.

■ The new live oral typhoid vaccine is also ignored in the Red Book, but in this case, health authority discretion is no help. Although typhoid immunization is included in the Red Book, no fee is payable for this route of vaccination (and it is even less financially attractive because no payment can be made under paragraph 44.5).

■ The introduction of active immunization against hepatitis A has left some health authorities paying only one higher-rate fee and others paying a lower fee for the first dose, a higher fee for the second dose and a further higher fee for the booster 6–12 months later. Although the single dose vaccine has led to a fee structure that is simpler, with the initial dose regarded as a B fee and the booster as a B fee, there is still the same payment problem in relation to the paediatric vaccine.

■ Some inner city health authorities will pay fees for hepatitis B immunization for all at-risk groups, on the basis that this work is being undertaken according to a community physician's recommendation.

BASIC ADULT IMMUNIZATION

Tetanus and polio

A significant proportion of the UK population is not immune from these diseases; this is, therefore, an area in which good preventative medicine can boost practice income.

Tetanus

The Green Book states unequivocally that every adult should have had a complete primary course of immunization against tetanus. Although the vaccine has been in use since the late 1930s, it was not until the mid 1950s that it was used on the civilian population as part of a primary course of immunization given to a limited number of young children. It was made nationally available in 1961. Therefore, a section of the UK population is still 'at risk' and, therefore, requires a primary course of immunization. All patients should be offered this, unless:

■ they were born after 1961 (because some people born after the mid-1950s may have been immunized, which should be checked)

■ there is a specific history or a record of a completed primary course

■ they have been in the armed forces during some period since 1938

■ they have received a tetanus course following an accident.

A full primary course earns item of service fees, as well as payments for personal administration of the vaccine itself. This income should more than compensate for the time taken to identify those at risk who should be called for immunization.

Two tetanus boosters should be given after the primary course, at 10-yearly intervals, each attracting the higher-rate B fee. Although this is sometimes followed by regular 10-yearly boosters, these probably confer no added immunity to someone who has had the primary course and two boosters, unless administered at the time of an injury.

Polio

The same fee structure applied to a primary course of polio immunizations; however, the patient should be either under 40 years of age or at risk of contracting the disease from an immunized child's nappy.

Boosters given to school leavers or for travel immunization also attract a fee.

PERSONALLY ADMINISTERED IMMUNIZATION

This scheme applies only to England and Wales and pays GPs for personally administering injectable immunizations to patients. Although it is termed 'personal administration', GPs can delegate the work to appropriate qualified staff, typically practice nurses acting on their behalf. Oral immunizations, such as those for polio and oral typhoid, are not included in the scheme. Since the change to centralized purchasing and supply of childhood immunizations, these are no longer available for purchase by GPs and are, therefore, excluded from this scheme. Diphtheria vaccine is also excluded if recommended for travel.

The scheme operates as follows.

▨ The GP buys the vaccine directly from a supplier or pharmacist.

▨ The practice administers the vaccine to the patient.

▨ A prescription is written on form FP10 for the immunization given.

▨ At the end of each month, all FP10s are sent to the Prescription Pricing Authority, together with form FP34D. (This is an entirely different procedure from sending in the FP73 claim forms, because FP34Ds are not sent to health authorities.)

▨ Six to 12 weeks later, the practice should receive reimbursement for the vaccines given, based on these costings:

— the cost of the vaccine

— a 10.5% on-cost allowance

— a container allowance

— a dispensing fee

— VAT.

The dispensing fee is reduced according to the total number of prescriptions submitted for payment. If the total is over 400, the payment for prescription is reduced; therefore prescriptions should be bundled separately for each individual partner so that fewer than 400 are submitted for each doctor and a reduction in the fee payable is avoided.

Most vaccine suppliers have a discount scheme, which allows further income to be earned from lower prices and VAT. The largest discounts tend to be in the most competitive areas. An example of how these discounts work is shown in Table 4.4.

It should be noted that this scheme applies to immunizations for which an item of service fee is not payable; therefore, hepatitis B, meningitis and Japanese B encephalitis vaccines are all included. Yellow fever is specifically excluded.

Running an immunization campaign in which personal administration fees can be earned

Influenza and pneumococcal immunization

Income under personal administration can be boosted by running seasonal campaigns against influenza for patients who are particu-

Table 4.4: Vaccine discounts

Expenditure		Income	
Havrix Mono	£21.60	Refund of cost price	£21.60
Less 12% discount	£2.60	On cost at 10.5%	£2.27
VAT on discounted price	£3.33	Container allowance	£0.04
		Dispensing fee	£0.97
		VAT	£3.78
Total	£22.30	Total	£28.66

larly vulnerable to this disease. The Department of Health advises that immunization should be offered annually to patients with diagnoses of:

▓ chronic respiratory disease (including asthma)

▓ chronic heart disease

▓ chronic renal failure

▓ endocrine disorders, such as diabetes

▓ immunosuppression.

It should also be noted that the elderly are at greater risk of the disease and that immunization is particularly recommended for residents of old people's homes, nursing homes and other long-stay institutions.

Many practices organize major immunization campaigns each autumn to protect those at risk, and, in some areas, these can cover up to 10% of a practice's patients. These campaigns can ensure that:

▓ patients are offered protection, helping to reduce mortality and morbidity

▓ the spread of an epidemic can be limited, thereby reducing the potentially heavy work-load that might otherwise be experienced by a practice

▓ the partners themselves and the practice staff are protected against influenza

▓ extra income is earned for the practice.

Closely related to influenza immunization is protection against Pneumococcus. This is because many patients at risk of influenza infection are also at risk of contracting pneumococcal pneumonia. The Green Book recommends that this immunization be given to the same risk groups as for influenza. In addition, it is indicated for patients with poor splenic function, i.e. those with:

▓ homozygous sickle cell disease

▓ asplenia or severe dysfunction of the spleen.

Influenza and pneumococcal immunizations can often be given to the same patient at the same time. However, unlike the vaccine for influenza, pneumococcal vaccine must be given only once, except to asplenic patients.

The only financial disadvantages to using this scheme for a course of immunization are that they are not eligible for payment on form FP73 and that patients cannot, therefore, be charged a private fee for the vaccination (Table 4.5).

However, a benefit is that, if the GP personally administers the immunization, the patient does not have to pay a prescription charge.

Table 4.5: Vaccine payments

Vaccine	FP73	Personal administration*	Private fee*
Hepatitis A	Yes	Yes	No
Hepatitis B	No	Yes	Yes
Tetanus	Yes	Yes	No
Polio	Yes	No	No
Typhoid Vi	Yes	Yes	No
– Oral	No	No	Yes
– Whole cell	Yes	Yes	No
Cholera	Yes	Yes	Yes, for certificate
Yellow fever	No	No	Yes, and for certificate
Meningitis – AC Vax	No	Yes	Yes
– Mengivac (AC)	No	Yes	Yes
Rabies	Yes	Yes	Yes
Japanese B encephalitis	No	Yes	Yes
Tick-borne encephalitis	No	Yes	Yes
Influenza	No	Yes	No
Pneumococcus	No	Yes	No

*A GP cannot charge a private fee for the vaccine and claim for personal administration, nor can an NHS prescription for the vaccine be written. However, the doctor can charge for certificates in all cases.

5

Obtaining and storing vaccines

How a practice obtains its vaccines depends on:

- the type of vaccine and its licence
- the type of immunization service it runs
- whether or not it is a dispensing practice
- where the practice is located
- its policy and philosophy.

These factors influence a practice's choice of supplier, bearing in mind that most practices will wish to earn some income from purchasing and administering vaccines.

TYPES OF VACCINE

Childhood immunization

In recent years, a central source of supply has provided all childhood immunization vaccines. Although there were initially many problems with this centralized supply, especially because it started when MMR vaccine was being introduced, its operation has considerably improved. Nevertheless, it has taken a long time for the centralized supply to reach acceptable standards. The introduction of Hib caused a repetition of the problems associated with MMR, and vaccine shortages hindered the 'catch-up' programme that the government was actively promoting.

The supply system has now been further changed. Whereas health authorities were previously supplying vaccines through hospital pharmacies, distribution is now provided by an independent company, Farillon. It has introduced regular deliveries of vaccines to practices, and although these are still somewhat infrequent, its service is gradually expanding. Unfortunately, deliveries are normally fortnightly, or even monthly, which means that it is difficult to obtain extra supplies if stocks are unexpectedly depleted.

In general, vaccine shortages are ultimately caused by poor central planning by Departments of Health prior to introducing new vaccines. Although memories may be fading, those GPs who experienced the difficulties associated with the introduction of MMR and Hib will not have forgotten their frustration at the time. Another problem with central supply is that it reduces the capacity of practices to respond promptly to local problems. For example, when two out of the three MMR vaccines were withdrawn because of possible side-effects, GPs were first informed of this decision through the media, and it was virtually impossible to get hold of the only remaining MMR vaccine. The income of many practices was adversely affected because they could not meet their immunization targets; they will recall the disastrous impact of reluctant parents turning up at the surgery for their children's injection only to be told that no vaccines were available.

In spite of its unproven record, a centralized supply is now an integral part of immunization policy, and new vaccines will be distributed through this system. From the profession's viewpoint, this development is not wholly welcome because many GPs prefer to purchase their own vaccines, not only because this arrangement contributes to practice income, but also because it ensures that individual practices can exercise more control over supply and the level of stock.

General vaccines

For other vaccines, there are various methods of supply, and which of these is used depends on the practice's preferences.

Writing a prescription for the vaccine

This is uncomplicated; a prescription is written for each patient prior to a return visit to receive the immunization. Patients take their prescription to a pharmacist, obtain the vaccine and bring it to the surgery for the nurse to administer.

Advantages include:

- its intrinsic simplicity
- the lack of a need to keep vaccine in stock
- the lack of problems associated with refrigerated storage
- the pharmacists being responsible for prompt supply of the vaccine and for ensuring that it has not expired
- the nurse only being responsible for its administration, because the doctor is actually prescribing the vaccine
- saving of NHS money, because patients pay a prescription charge for the vaccine
- the lack of risk of being left with useless and expensive stock, such as last year's influenza vaccine.

Disadvantages include:

- cumbersome administration, because the doctor has to write a prescription and the patient cannot book the appointment until the vaccine has been dispensed
- inflexibility; for example, if a patient fails to mention a particular stop on an international journey, or discloses that he or she has never had a primary course of vaccination, no stock is available in the practice to make last minute adjustments
- patients paying prescription charges, which can make the service comparatively expensive

▓ the loss of potentially significant practice income from the personal administration scheme if a substantial number of immunizations is being given

▓ a lack of incentive for practices to develop their immunization service.

Purchasing vaccine

This arrangement involves buying vaccine from an independent supplier. Most non-dispensing practices cannot obtain their supplies from a pharmaceutical wholesaler, who could otherwise offer an excellent service, combining both attractive discounts and prompt delivery. Other alternative suppliers include:

▓ a local pharmacist who is conveniently located and can provide prompt and frequent deliveries. However, buying from this source means paying a premium unless the pharmacist makes his or her own purchases at heavily discounted prices and passes on some of these savings. Nevertheless, a pharmacist will probably accept returns of unused stock (apart from influenza vaccines) and will even store vaccines for the practice, allowing it to draw off its requirements in small batches

▓ a manufacturer; most pharmaceutical companies are willing to supply products directly to practices at a discount, depending on the vaccine and on market conditions.

Unlicenced vaccine

This category includes some less commonly used travel vaccines, for example Japanese B encephalitis and tick-borne encephalitis vaccines. These can be bought in the same way as licenced vaccines: through the pharmacist or directly from a manufacturer. However, because they are not on general licence but are supplied instead only to named patients, different regulations apply to their purchase. In particular, the patient's name has to be stated at the time of ordering. There should be no difficulty in ordering these vaccines from any source, and no medicolegal problems should arise from their administration if they are given for a valid condition and satisfactory records are kept.

BUYING VACCINES

The decision whether to purchase vaccines and the choice of a supplier depends on several factors. The first decision is to assess which of the factors listed below are particularly important:

■ price

■ delivery

■ stock back-up

■ credit

■ information services

■ patient and practice services

■ reliability.

For example, whereas price may be a key factor in one practice, another practice with limited storage facilities may prefer to pay more to a supplier who delivers small quantities frequently. Another practice with cash flow problems and a substantial overdraft may prefer to pay more to a supplier who offers credit.

Price

This factor is obviously important to many practices. The actual cost of the vaccine will be affected by several variables. The more a practice buys, the more ability it has to negotiate a higher discount; thus, its negotiating position will be further enhanced if it is a large practice. Price also depends on competition between suppliers: suppliers of a vaccine (e.g. active hepatitis A) from a monopoly source do not have to engage in price competition. In contrast, there is intense competition between manufacturers of influenza vaccine, leading to substantial discounts, which can be as much as 25–30% when a new manufacturer enters the field.

When negotiating the most competitive price, a practice should take account of the following issues.

▓ The size of its order will affect the price offered.

▓ If a manufacturer offers a range of vaccines, buying from across the range allows the negotiation of higher discounts on all the antigens purchased. It may be advisable to highlight the total amount being spent on the company's products, rather than the number of doses of each vaccine. Competition is important; thus, a vaccine such as influenza, with which there is intense competition, is likely to attract higher discounts. A practice can use its annual influenza vaccine order to beat down prices of other vaccines across a particular manufacturer's range.

▓ If a practice remains loyal to a manufacturer, this should be rewarded in the service and/or price it receives.

Because smaller practices are often disadvantaged with respect to price, purchasing consortia can help. Several practices within the same area can benefit from buying their vaccines jointly. Obviously, they need to decide which vaccines to use. These consortia of practices have two main strengths.

▓ The size of their order means that they should receive substantial discounts and be able to negotiate with a more senior person in the sales hierarchy, leading to faster decisions and more initiative and flexibility.

▓ Who ever gets a consortium's order will effectively 'clean up' in that area, which is an added incentive to the company.

Delivery

It is advisable not to keep too much stock because:

▓ less refrigeration storage space is required

▓ there is less risk of losing stock because of power failure, accidental damage or poor stock control

▓ less capital, which would otherwise be available to the practice, is tied up in stock.

Low stock levels can only be achieved if the supplier's delivery arrangements are responsive, prompt and efficient. If this is so, a practice can plan its orders in the certainty that extra stock will be supplied as and when required. The faster the response time, the better. However much a practice may pride itself on being efficient, organized and computerized, unanticipated situations occur in which something goes wrong and vaccines are needed quickly. Any company that offers same day or next day delivery may well be offering the practice both financial and organizational benefits. Remote practices, on islands or in areas with adverse weather conditions, need to ensure that the delivery service being offered is guaranteed.

Stock back-up

It is possible to get the best of both worlds by negotiating discounts on the basis of a year's total vaccine supply, thereby boosting the quantity ordered while drawing off the numbers actually used as and when required, thus minimizing actual refrigerated stock. This facility offers real advantages for many practices.

Credit

This is usually most important when interest rates are high and the cost of any overdraft is also correspondingly high. The longer the timescale over which the practice is allowed to pay bills, the longer the time it has to use the vaccines, write and send off prescriptions and receive payments. Fortunately, the Prescription Pricing Authority is reducing the time its payments take to arrive from 12 to six weeks, which should ease some cash flow pressures. In effect, extended credit means that the practice is getting the worthwhile bonus of an interest-free loan.

Information services

Information about immunization is important, and easy access to it can improve the practice's service. Paper-based or computerized information (on disk or on line) is attractive to some practices.

Patient and practice services

Many pharmaceutical companies have well established services. They often produce attractive patient record cards, recall systems, posters, handbooks and travel advice sheets. These reduce practice costs and help the practice to market its service. Some companies offer advice on immunization protocols and provide educational material, such as hand-books and other written material, for staff and patients. These support services can be of particular value to a practice when it is first setting up an immunization service.

Reliability

Continuity of supply is particularly important. The problem with vaccines is that they are organic and cultivated, rather than manufactured chemicals: they are the product not of a chemical synthesis but of a culture of living organisms. This means that supply cannot suddenly be increased through a chemical process. Because of these constraints on output, reliability is especially important—a sudden batch failure or product withdrawal can create great difficulties in the search for an alternative supply. Past reliability of a manufacturer should give some indication of future reliability, but it is never easy to predict the future.

Having considered the factors above, a practice policy can be drawn up to provide a basis for negotiations with potential suppliers and to help to choose the one that most closely matches its requirements.

STOCK CONTROL

Vaccines are expensive and perishable, many having very short shelf lives. Because they are composed of biological material, they are sensitive to maltreatment and incorrect storage. Any vaccine stored incorrectly or beyond its expiry date has to be disposed of, which represents a direct financial loss for the practice. If disposal becomes necessary, it may indicate a serious flaw in the organization of the practice's service. The practice should identify why it has happened and introduce changes to ensure that it does not happen again. It is essential to avoid such losses, through the use of several procedures.

Delegation

A specific person should be in charge of stock control, usually a practice nurse. By allocating this responsibility to one person, it can be ensured that the tasks involved are carried out regularly and conscientiously.

Training

The designated person must know how to control stock. When imparting knowledge, it is important to emphasize the financial and clinical implications of wasted stock and to spell out procedures that need to be followed to prevent it happening.

Checking stock levels

If negotiations with the supplier have been successful, it should be possible to run the service with a low stock level. Although this lowers the risk of waste, it can mean that the practice will run out of an essential vaccine. Each practice has to decide on the size of its stock level, but it is vital to check regularly that correct amounts of vaccines are held. Again, if rapid delivery times have been agreed with the supplier, vaccines can be replenished quickly.

Stock rotation

It is essential that vaccines are put straight into a refrigerator when they arrive and to ensure that stock is rotated, so that vaccines with the earlier expiry dates are readily available and used first. To help stock rotation, it is useful to write the expiry date boldly on boxes of vaccines.

Expiry dates

The practice should confirm the life of the vaccines that are ordered and that these are reasonable. Although influenza vaccine normally has a nine-month life, it can only be used during one season; other vaccines should have a two- or three-year life span.

Childhood immunizations cannot be bought directly but only ordered through the Department of Health's central distribution system. This has the advantage of avoiding any financial risk if stock control is not implemented. Indeed, because of GPs' lack of confidence in the Department of Health's ability to ensure vaccine supplies when new agents are introduced or others withdrawn, practices may benefit from holding excess stock. If a vaccine expires and has to be thrown away, there is no loss to the practice, whereas if a practice is short of a vaccine and a completing dose has to be postponed, there is a real chance that substantial practice income could be lost because targets are not reached.

STORAGE

Because vaccines are delicate, live materials, correct refrigerated storage is vital. Temperature must be controlled from when the vaccine first arrives at the practice until it is administered to the patient. Warming can lead to loss of potency, while too low a temperature can cause freezing and even more severe damage.

Receiving the vaccines

Most suppliers dispatch vaccines via experienced carriers, and the vaccines should be dated and time stamped. Packaging always carries instructions on perishability, and before accepting delivery, staff should ensure that the time shown on the package has not been exceeded.

When the package arrives, it should be unpacked and immediately put in the refrigerator. Although this task sounds simple enough, all too often a receptionist accepts the package and puts it down whilst carrying on with his or her normal duties or while being distracted by a demanding patient, a difficult phone call or even a stressed doctor. In these circumstances, a vaccine could spend some time by a radiator or in sunlight and be damaged before being placed in a refrigerator.

Training is important, so that reception staff know that whoever accepts the package takes responsibility for handing it to the practice nurse or unpacking and storing its contents him- or herself.

Storing vaccines

Although any commercial refrigerator is adequate, there are specialized products with a higher specification, including refinements such as internal fans to equalize the temperature. The Department of Health publishes advice on vaccine storage and a list of refrigerators approved by the government's buying agency[3].

A refrigerator should:

▥ maintain a temperature of 0–4°C, irrespective of the external temperature

▥ be large enough to cope with the practice's stock and range of vaccines; sufficient room should be allowed for the annual influenza vaccine stock

▥ have a thermometer that can be read from the outside without opening the door

▥ have a minimum/maximum thermometer to ensure that parameters for safe storage are continually maintained

---

[3]Fact sheet reference 2250/1050pc+/5-18/cd/1; Government buying agency, Tel: 0151 227 4262 ext. 2246.

▓ be wired directly into a fused spur, so that a switch cannot be accidentally turned off or a plug pulled out

▓ be lockable

▓ be self-defrosting to increase efficiency but designed so that the temperature does not exceed the maximum for safe vaccine storage during the defrosting cycle

▓ have a door that cannot be accidentally left open with a bleep or alarm system installed.

Transferring the vaccine

Problems arise when a vaccine is transferred from the refrigerator, because it can be damaged by a rise in temperature. Opportunistic immunization programmes may involve leaving vaccines for each surgery session out on the doctor's desk; this should be done only if the life of the vaccine away from the refrigerator has been checked with the manufacturer; otherwise, its potency could be lost.

In general, whenever a vaccine is removed from the refrigerator, it should be stored in a cool bag, unless it is to be used immediately. Cool bags are widely available, as are the large, rigid cool boxes that are so useful for keeping drinks cold at Test Matches, Henley or Ascot! They should have an 'ice' block placed in them to keep the temperature down, but the vaccine should be kept away from the block itself in case it is actually frozen. The bags or boxes can be used for transferring a vaccine to a branch surgery, school immunization session, old people's home or wherever immunizations are to be given. They should also be used if the refrigerator is being defrosted, to ensure that the vaccines are kept within their normal temperature range.

6

Private immunization services

The NHS provides GPs with most of their income from immunizations. Together with other related NHS payments and staff reimbursements, it is readily apparent that providing NHS immunization services makes good sense. Against this background, some practices are reluctant to consider running private immunization services—surely, if a practice runs its NHS services well, how can there be further benefits from private services? Can they be expected to repay the time, effort and enthusiasm required to run them successfully? This may be a worthy and cautious view, but there are several reasons why practices should assess the feasibility of a private immunization service. Common arguments for and against running private immunization services include the following.

▓ 'They involve private clinics.' Although this may be the popular image, private clinics are in fact a specialized activity within the private sector and do not need to be run in the generality of NHS practices. In the context of NHS general practice, the term 'private immunization services' refers to a range of comparatively routine activities, such as certification and the sale of particular products and services, which can be easily integrated into the normal day-to-day work of an NHS practice.

▓ 'They are already being run elsewhere.' It is very rare to find a practice that does not charge a fee for countersigning passport forms, giving yellow fever vaccine or certifying fitness to travel.

Therefore, any expansion of these services should fit quite easily into a practice's normal working arrangements and procedures.

▣ 'Earnings from this source are outside average net remuneration.' NHS immunization services (apart from the higher target premiums) are included in GPs' average net pay. This means that as more individual fees are earned from NHS work, the fees are liable to be reduced to contain average GP earnings at the intended level. Private earnings obviously lie outside this system; the more the profession earns, the more it actually keeps.

▣ 'They can be as narrow or as broad in their range as the doctor wishes.' Doctors can limit the level of their involvement in providing private services to whatever amount they wish.

▣ 'They can enhance the doctor's NHS service.' The quality expected when patients are paying directly is often higher, which can stimulate improved standards in a practice's NHS service.

▣ 'They can add to the doctor's pension.' As with other private earnings, they can be used to buy added pension rights while retaining membership of the NHS superannuation scheme.

OTHER SERVICES LINKED TO IMMUNIZATION

If a practice has a thriving travel immunization service, there will be further opportunities to increase private income from other activities related to travel. These represent a natural spin-off from providing high-quality NHS services. The more that patients are attracted to the immunization service or are identified as requiring immunization through opportunistic screening, the more likely they are to need other private services related to travel.

Certification

▣ Vaccination certificates. International vaccination certificates only apply to yellow fever and cholera vaccines. The cost of the yellow fever certificate is usually included in the total fee charged to the immunization. The certificate itself is the sole remaining justification for the cholera vaccination; apart from this use, the vaccination is generally regarded as ineffective. The Green Book states that cholera vaccination should not be required of any traveller and that it is indicated neither in the control of outbreaks nor in the management of contacts of imported cases.

▨ Health certificates. There is increasing demand for these from:

— travel insurance companies, who will not insure elderly or high-risk patients without a doctor's letter

— tour operators, for example, Club Med insist on a 'freedom from infection' certificate for children using their facilities

— cruise ships, which often require their own medical form to be completed.

The BMA recommends a set scale of fees for this work.

Private prescriptions

In early 1995 the Department of Health ruled that drugs for malaria prophylaxis would no longer be prescribable on a normal prescription form FP10. Although this has meant that patients will have to purchase their own drugs from the pharmacist there are some antimalarials, notably mefloquine, that are only available by prescription and so the intending traveller will have to request a private prescription.

The regulations allow a charge to be made for issuing a private prescription and at present the BMA recommends a fee of £6.00; though in practice charges vary.

In addition to malaria prophylactics other drugs specifically prescribed for use abroad may have to be issued by private prescription and the same fee can be charged.

Passports

Many patients ask their GP to countersign a passport application. This is an additional source of income that carries its own risks. The recommended fee does not reflect the risk that unintentional mistakes can lead to a GP being prosecuted. This was highlighted recently when a GP was prosecuted for signing the passport application form of a patient who, while registered with the practice, had used a false name, which the GP subsequently confirmed on the form.

It is vital to check the following details: the patient's name, date of birth and date of registration; the patient's address; the date the patient was first seen by the doctor; and, finally, that the photograph resembles the patient.

Countersigning carries a great deal of responsibility; if in doubt, a passport application form should not be signed.

Examinations

There are various circumstances in which an examination or an extract from a patient's records is required for travel, for example for:

■ teenagers attending camps abroad or working on a kibbutz

■ the elderly

■ those with chronic disease.

In general, these should be treated as full examinations and charged at the normal rate; however, the option of extracting information from the patient's records for a lower fee may be appropriate.

Private immunizations

There are several vaccination courses that are not eligible for payment by the NHS. If this is the case, there are two ways of earning income from this work, which are:

■ personal administration (see Chapter 4); this is not available to GPs in Scotland or Northern Ireland

■ charging the patient for the vaccine and the fee for administering it.

The fee should cover the doctor or nurse's professional time when administering the immunization course. If this charge is made, the vaccine itself cannot be prescribed using form FP10 because this would mix NHS and private practice in the treatment of an NHS patient. Therefore, an additional charge has to be made to cover the cost of the vaccine itself.

Under this arrangement, the cost of a course of hepatitis B would be:

- £12.13 for the vaccine in the prefilled syringe form or £36.39 for a course of three injections

- £6.36 for VAT on the vaccine

- £18.50 for the private administration fee.

This makes a total of £61.25 for the course, which does not include any profit on the vaccine itself. It is, therefore, an expensive way of providing the service.

It is important to ensure that doctors do not mix private and NHS practice when providing a particular episode of treatment to an NHS patient. However, there is no reason why different approaches should be used for different vaccines; some can be given under the personal administration scheme and some can be charged for.

PRIVATE IMMUNIZATION CLINICS

As travel to exotic locations has increased, there are greater opportunities for practices to run private immunization clinics. Before doing so, a practice should decide at which market it is aiming its private services: is the service:

- a private vaccination service for patients on its NHS list?

- a private vaccination service for all patients?

- a comprehensive franchised private travel clinic?

There is some scope for running a comparatively small-scale service that attracts private patients from neighbouring practices for specific vaccines, such as yellow fever. However, once it is decided to develop the private service beyond the NHS practice, it usually expands to become a fully comprehensive private immunization service.

A practice can develop a private clinic either independently or in partnership with a commercial organization that franchises clinics, for example the British Airways travel clinics.

An example of a franchise clinic

British Airways requires a practice to satisfy several conditions before granting a franchise.

▓ Its premises must suit the purpose, having a well-decorated and adequately sized waiting area and reasonable parking facilities, and be accessible to public transport.

▓ Staff must meet the standards set by British Airways.

▓ The geographical area must be able to sustain an immunization clinic; a survey is undertaken jointly by the franchiser and franschisee to assess whether or not there will be sufficient demand to make the project viable.

▓ An IBM-compatible computer and modem must be acquired, together with a cash register, a refrigerator for storing vaccines and a photocopier.

The franchise lasts for about five years and involves a single fee of approximately £5000 (1995 value), in addition to the payment of 10% of the turnover of the clinic.

The advantage of this type of clinic to a practice is that it is buying in an established service that is widely known and well marketed; membership brings signs, supplies, information systems, training and marketing, and the practice receives continuing help in running its immunization service. Opportunities to obtain this franchise are limited by the level of demand for the service. Although a few practices have successfully embarked on this venture, it may not be suited to others.

Independent private clinics

Another alternative is developing a private service under a practice's own auspices. In doing so, the practice must consider carefully what kind of service it intends to provide by addressing the following issues.

▧ Clinic times—clinics should be held at time that attract private patients, i.e. there should be either early morning or late evening sessions on weekdays, together with Saturday morning or all-day sessions. The practice should then consider the potential staffing costs (extra staff and overtime payments) and also the need for a doctor to be present at the clinic during opening hours.

▧ Premises—is there enough space in the waiting room? Should there be a separate waiting area for private patients? Will the practice nurses' treatment room be sufficient or is extra room needed?

▧ Appointments—for clients to be attracted and retained, they have to get through easily on the telephone and will expect calls to be answered promptly. Thus extra costs may have to be incurred in installing new telephone lines and equipment and ensuring that staff are available to answer their enquiries.

▧ Staff—staff will have to work later, and extra personnel may be needed. In addition, if these clinics start to boost private earning to the extent that they are greater than 10% of total practice earnings, abatement of direct reimbursements will occur. (The same abatement also applies to direct reimbursements for premises.)

▧ Nursing—should an extra practice nurse be employed, or will the existing practice nurses work in the private clinic as part of their normal duties? If so will it be without extra payment or in return for extra pay?

▧ Equipment—although the practice may have a refrigerator, additional capacity may be needed for the clinic. The private clinic must have access to up-to-date immunization information, which is most easily obtained from a computerized database. This may require additional computer equipment and modems, a subscription to the information service and another telephone line.

▦ Stationery—there will be the cost of producing stationery for the clinic, including questionnaires, appointment cards and specialized record and note-taking systems. There is also the cost of printing patient advice leaflets.

▦ Training and education—normally this should already have been carried out for the NHS immunization service, but if it has not, it will certainly be required for a private service.

Financial considerations

It is important to estimate the costs and benefits of such a clinic. Fees must be set at a level that maintains profitability and covers costs, but they cannot vary greatly from those charged by neighbouring practices. Great care should be taken when calculating whether or not the clinic will be financially viable, including estimating the likely number of customers and the likely costs; from these estimates, the practice should try to assess whether or not all this effort will actually earn a profit.

Marketing

Marketing of immunization services is discussed in Chapter 10. It is important to consider how to attract customers to the clinic, given that most patients can receive the same vaccines from their GP for little, if any, charge. For this reason, the practice needs to assess how its private clinic can offer a significant advantage over local GP services. Obviously, convenient appointment times, a thorough and comprehensive service and providing a one-stop travel health shop are all factors that can encourage private patients to attend.

A good quality and highly efficient private travel service can lead to an improved standard of NHS service, but doctors must be vigilant about maintaining the crucial distinction between private and NHS services in relation to patients on their lists.

PROVIDING A SERVICE TO LOCAL COMPANIES

Some firms whose employees are involved in considerable international travel arrange for a local practice to meet their employees' travel needs. Therefore, it is worth investigating whether or not any local firms might be looking for this type of service.

To succeed a practice must be responsive to a companies' particular needs; these are probably similar to those of private patients, as described above, and include a convenient location and appointment times that suit the working day. Obviously, short notice travel may be commonplace, and the practice will need to be prepared to meet sudden demands for its services. When approaching companies, it should be stressed that the practice's immunization service can make savings for a firm (measured in terms of both cost and time) over and above its present arrangements for travel immunization.

Some firms may not have considered providing this service for employees travelling on official business. The practice may need to emphasize how illnesses contracted abroad can have potentially serious consequences for both the firm and its employees, as a result of prolonged sickness absence.

EQUIPMENT SALES

The sale of equipment to those travelling abroad can benefit both the practice and its private patients.

- It enables patients to receive advice on and buy their travel equipment.
- It reflects well on the professionalism and thoroughness of the service being offered.
- It provides additional income.

Travel health advice is an integral part of the overall service; it is appropriate, therefore, for travel packs and equipment to augment fact sheets and leaflets. Patients can be advised on which equipment is best suited to their needs. Moreover, as failing prophylaxis becomes more common, precautions against mosquito bites are becoming more important in preventing infection from this parasite; by having netting, insect repellents and sprays available, the advice given can be easily translated into action.

Equipment that can be sold to private patient travellers includes:

■ first-aid kits

■ anti-HIV sterile kits

■ malaria tablets

■ water sterilizing tablets and equipment

■ mosquito nets

■ insect repellents

■ sunscreens.

The person who is responsible for ordering and monitoring vaccine stocks should also check the stock of travel equipment and packs for private patients. However, decisions on range and stock level should be made after consultation with the doctors.

There are a number of companies producing these packs, some of which are listed below, and skills acquired when negotiating vaccine prices could be deployed when buying these kits.

■ Nomad Ltd
  3 Turnpike Lane
  London N8 ODA
  Tel: 0181 889 7814

■ Lifesystems
  4 Mercury House
  Calleva Park
  Aldermaston
  Berkshire
  Tel: 01734 811433

■ Homeway Medical
  Littleton
  Winchester SO22 6QS
  Tel: 01962 881526

7

Medicolegal aspects of immunization

As our society has become increasingly litigious, attitudes towards cause and responsibility have also changed. When the professional image of medicine was far more potent than its capacity to treat disease, there was little desire to attribute blame for adverse events: fate was seen to be the cause, and those who gave treatment had done all that they could. The public was both more ignorant of medical matters and more trusting, allowing the health professions to adopt a paternalistic and even patronizing manner towards patients.

The public is now more aware of its health and its illnesses and makes increased demand on its doctors. Patients expect explanations about their condition, the treatment proposed and any side-effects, and even may wish to participate in decisions about treatment.

Most patients' contact with GPs is initiated by the patients themselves; they perceive a problem that requires a GP's help and ask for a consultation or home visit to obtain advice and assistance. An underlying ethos of paternalism inevitably permeates GPs' relations with their patients, however much they aim to ensure that these are based on the principle of equality.

Immunization, however, usually occurs in a very different context.

▨ It is often initiated by a GP practice, health authority or hospital accident and emergency department:

— a health authority in the case of childhood immunizations

— a practice for routine adult and travel immunizations

— a hospital accident and emergency department for tetanus courses.

▦ It is usually administered to patients who are in normal health; thus, side-effects are regarded in very negative terms, whereas the lack of any side-effects will not be regarded at all positively.

▦ It is apparently given for a negative rather than a positive reason; nothing is perceived as being done that is immediately and directly helpful to the patient, in contrast, for example, to treating asthma or eradicating an infection. (Patients do not write to thank their GPs for helping them to avoid tetanus and typhoid during their holidays!)

▦ It is given to patients who may (sometimes justifiably) fear adverse reactions; some vaccines generate a real fear of brain damage or other adverse events.

It is important to counter any fears and uncertainties by ensuring that a high standard of service is provided. There are some well-known areas in which problems may be encountered, which can be largely avoided by ensuring that procedures and protocols are understood, agreed and followed.

CONSENT

This can be either implied or expressed verbally or in writing. Implied consent means that it is not actually expressed but can be inferred from the context in which the treatment is being provided. For example, a patient comes for an immunization, rolls up a sleeve and allows an injection to take place; in these circumstances, it may be assumed that he or she has given implied consent for the vaccine to be administered, on the condition the entire procedure has been done voluntarily. Indeed, it could be argued that the request for an appointment and attendance at surgery for the vaccination in themselves imply consent.

Expressed consent can be given verbally or in writing. Either can be equally valid, particularly if verbal consent is witnessed. Obviously, written consent is much easier to prove.

However consent is obtained, the ultimate legal test is whether or not the consent is knowingly given, i.e. whether or not the patient has been informed, in broad terms, what the procedure entails. Thus, this consent is specific to the proposed procedure and not to any other. This means that if a patient consents to an influenza vaccine being administered, his or her consent is limited to that procedure, and a GP cannot proceed to give a Pneumococcus vaccine in addition, without additional specific consent.

The issue of consent is complicated by the lack of firm rulings on the matter. This uncertainty is reflected in practice by inconsistent approaches; on some occasions, or in some practices, written expressed consent is sought, while in others, implied consent is assumed to be sufficient. These variations in day-to-day practice actually serve to help GPs should they have to defend their actions (or inaction) in court. Because there is no definitive ruling under English law on the notion of informed consent, what should be said to patients when warning them of the possible effects and problems of the treatment that they are undergoing is judged according to what is known as the 'Bolam Test'. This is based on a 1957 legal case concerning negligence; it amounts to the proposition that if a body of qualified practitioners in a particular field accepts what is being done as being reasonable (whatever the majority believes), the action itself is not negligent. The corollary of this is that informed consent may be obtained in a manner that conforms to that which is considered reasonable by a minority of the profession. If the information given to patients, and the extent to which side-effects have been discussed, falls into this range of 'reasonableness' there should be no grounds for legal action on the issue of consent. However, it should also be noted that:

▨ if a doctor or nurse is specifically asked about any risks of side-effects, such questions should be answered

▨ if there is a common risk or side-effect, however minor (e.g. local redness and erythema after a tetanus immunization) the patient should be told

▨ if there is a risk, however minor, of a rare but serious side-effect (e.g. encephalitis after a pertussis vaccination) the patient should be warned.

It is undoubtedly preferable, wherever practicable, to obtain written consent; ideally, it should be signed by the patient after he or she has had the opportunity to discuss possible side-effects. Although this cautious approach can be time-consuming and bureaucratic, it can be simplified by incorporating the procedure of obtaining written consent into a protocol that specifies how consent has to be obtained and how the patient should be given written information about the vaccine and its possible side-effects. If a protocol is adopted, the only reference that needs to be included in the patient's notes is 'advised per protocol'.

An additional benefit of such protocols is that they enhance verbal consent. If the protocol specifies what information is given and how consent is obtained, an entry in the patient's notes, recording that it has been followed, is most helpful should there be any subsequent litigation. It would be difficult for a potential litigant to claim successfully that consent had not been forthcoming if the notes showed that the patient had been informed and consent had been obtained according to an established procedure. If virtually all practices used protocols, the legally acceptable standard of practice would be raised, and all practices would be expected to use them. Any failure to do so would constitute a failure to practise at a reasonable standard, leaving a practice open to the charge of negligence. Obviously, these higher standards are to be encouraged, but the profession should be wary of making a rod for its own back.

Children's consent

In most cases, parental consent should be sought for childhood immunization. If a parent is not available, consent should be sought from someone who has legal charge of the child. Problems can arise if a parent is not present when the procedure is being undertaken, for example when a grandparent brings the child for immunization. In such cases, if the parent is aware that the child is being brought to the surgery for immunization, implied consent can be assumed to have been given. Moreover, the grandparent can be assumed to be acting as the parents' agent for these purposes, and is thereby able to give consent.

Children can give their own consent if they are old enough. The famous Gillick case established a ruling that there is no lower age limit to consent; once children are old enough to understand and make a decision about treatment, they can give consent. The 1994 measles/rubella immunization campaign encouraged older children to request vaccination; although it would have been appropriate to accept their consent if they were over the age of 16, or seek the parents' consent for under-16s, a child would be able to consent to the vaccine were he or she capable of understanding the reasons for immunization and its side-effects.

It is reassuring to note that for an action for damages to be successful, actual damages must have occurred and been proven. Thus, even if consent were not properly obtained, damages must have resulted for legal action to succeed.

CONTRAINDICATIONS

There is a duty of care to the patient, which means that the standard of professional practice must be acceptable; in particular this behoves GPs to:

- give accurate and relevant information about immunization. Patients seeking advice should expect to receive clear and accurate information on such matters as immunization requirements for travel. The person giving the advice should be in a position to justify it by reference to authoritative sources

- know the contraindications

- be able to inform patient about any side-effects.

There is much concern about childhood immunizations and their adverse reactions; anyone giving these must know their contraindications and cautions and be able to discuss these with worried parents.

Again, a protocol can specify the circumstances when vaccines may be given, thereby helping to eliminate many of these potential risks.

COMPLIANCE

This is largely the patient's responsibility. The practice itself has a limited role.

▧ Patients should be told when their next immunization is due, and this fact should be noted in their records. This ensures that responsibility for completing the course lies firmly with the patient, rather than the doctor.

▧ It is useful to give the patient a record card, and to specify that this should be done in the practice's protocol, so that there is firm, written evidence that this duty has been discharged.

▧ If reminder letters are sent, a record that this has been done should be included either on the computer or in the patient's notes. A record should also be made of any recalls by telephone.

One important aspect of patient compliance concerns refusal to comply with childhood, travel or routine immunization. Deliberate refusals can be covered by the practice protocol.

▧ The fact that advice was given should be noted, together with the source of the advice.

▧ A patient's refusal to accept advice should also be recorded.

▧ It should be explained to the patient that he or she runs a risk of contracting the disease if the advice is not heeded.

The refusal to accept childhood immunization has important clinical consequences. However, care must be taken to respect consent. Although detailed explanations and intensive persuasion may come from doctors and practice staff, great care must be taken to ensure that there is no coercion. Consent obtained under any kind of duress is legally invalid.

COMPETENCE

Practice nurses often give immunizations; how they do so and their competence to do so can have important medicolegal consequences. Certain conditions must be met before nurses should be allowed to immunize; these are stated in the Green Book.

▧ The nurse must be prepared to be professionally accountable for this work.

▓ The nurse must have received adequate training and be competent in all aspects of immunization, including knowing the contraindications to specific vaccines.

▓ Adequate training must have been given in the recognition and treatment of anaphylaxis.

Nurses employed by GPs should work to agreed protocols that include these conditions.

Another important legal matter concerns the restrictions on nurses' ability to prescribe. The Medicines Act of 1968 remains the main point of reference regarding nurse prescribing. Although new legislation has been recently introduced (the Medicinal Products: Prescription by Nurses etc. Act 1992), which allows nurses to prescribe from a limited range of products, it has not yet been implemented, other than on a pilot basis. In any case, it is unlikely that vaccines will be included in the nurses' formulary.

At present, nurses may not prescribe vaccines or administer them without their having previously been prescribed by a doctor. The United Kingdom Central Council for Nurses, Midwives and Health Visitors (UKCC) has also issued advisory guidelines that reinforce this position.

It is essential that nurses only give immunizations in circumstances in which they are not vulnerable to legal action, which means that one of the following conditions should be met.

▓ There should be a specific instruction in the patient's notes.

▓ The vaccine has been dispensed on an FP10 prescription.

▓ There is a patient-specific protocol arrangement.

▓ There is a group protocol arrangement.

Even if one of the above conditions is fulfilled, it is nevertheless important to ensure that the nurse is confident and competent to follow these instructions.

Instruction in the patient's notes

It is entirely proper for a practice nurse to give an immunization or vaccination by following a GP's written instruction in the patient's notes. This written instruction could be computer-generated, providing the entry has been made by a GP. Of course, the nurse still has to ensure that normal safeguards are followed, namely that:

- the patient's identity matches the name on the notes that include the instruction

- the dosage and route of administration requested are correct

- the patient is receiving no other drugs that would be incompatible with the immunization or vaccination requested

- the patient has consented to the administration

- an accurate and contemporaneous record of the administration is made in the patient's notes.

Dispensation on an FP10 prescription

A nurse administering a vaccine is fully covered by a prescription issued by a GP, if the nurse exercises reasonable care.

Patient-specific protocol

A patient-specific protocol details the vaccine to be given to the patient, the dose, the route of administration and the circumstances in which it should be given, i.e. the instructions given at the beginning of any course of vaccinations that cover the administration of subsequent doses. Obviously, this approach is of limited use and can be extremely repetitive.

Group protocol

A group protocol is by far the most useful way of ensuring that all medicolegal risks are covered with respect to all staff involved in immunization. It is a written agreement authorizing the nurse to administer a specific group of immunizations to certain patients under clearly defined circumstances.

For a nurse to be able to feel confident of the cover of a group protocol, the UKCC guidance requires certain conditions to be fulfilled:

▓ it must be agreed by all the doctors working in a particular setting

▓ it should specify the circumstances in which the medicine can be administered

▓ one of the doctors should be responsible for instructing the nurse about the medicine.

Protocols do not absolve the nurse from responsibility for ensuring that the patient is fit to receive the vaccine and that it is administered in the correct manner.

Protocols also help to define the liability of doctors for the actions of their nurses. According to English law, an employer is vicariously liable for the negligent actions or omissions of his or her employees. Against this background, protocols define what the employer requires of the employees; any departure from a protocol would be entirely the responsibility of the nurse. Contracts of employment should stipulate that employees must comply with any protocols laid down by the practice.

There is a duty on doctors to ensure that anyone to whom they delegate a task is competent to perform that task. The General Medical Council Blue Book states this quite clearly in paragraph 42 of 'Professional conduct and discipline: fitness to practise': 'The Council recognizes and welcomes the growing contribution made to health care by nurses and other persons . . . but a doctor who delegates treatment or other procedures must be satisfied the person to whom they are delegated is competent to carry them out.'

This is not just a matter of professional discipline; ensuring the competence of staff is also covered by the GP's terms of service, which specify that 'A doctor shall, before employing any person to assist him, . . satisfy him or herself that the person is suitably qualified and competent'. This has important consequences, because it means that failure of GPs to satisfy themselves that these requirements have been met can lead to complaints being made and all the unpleasantness of a formal health authority medical service committee hearing.

An example of the group protocol would be:

Immunization and Vaccination (Model Agreement)

Name . . . .

The above named nurse has been fully instructed in the administration of the following vaccines and immunization procedures:

Cholera vaccine   Hepatitis A vaccine
Influenza vaccine   Hepatitis B vaccine
Polio vaccine   MMR vaccine (measles, mumps, rubella)
Tetanus vaccine   Rabies vaccine
. . . (other)   Typhoid vaccine
                                   . . . (other)

She is competent in the administration of the vaccines and has a good knowledge and understanding of indications and their use, recommended dosages, contraindications and side effects.

She has also had adequate training in the recognition and treatment of anaphylaxis and an anaphylactic shock pack is readily available and frequently checked.

The above named immunizations should only be administered in the presence of another responsible adult who could assist in case of emergency.

I/we . . . . (name of general practitioners) therefore give authorization for . . . .

to administer these vaccines as prescribed within this protocol and in accordance with the current Department of Health Guidelines.

Signed . . . . (general practitioners)

Date . . . .

I . . . . hereby agree that I have received adequate instruction for the above procedures and am willing to perform this duty.

Signed . . . .   Date . . . .

8

Business planning

Traditionally, general practice has developed according to the enthusiasms and interests of individual practitioners. Changes have often been implemented in a somewhat amateur and diffident style and have depended on a wide variety of motives. Thus, the sheer diversity of GPs and their interests have often meant that practice developments are the results of the enthusiasm, sheer personal commitment or dominance of an individual partner, rather than deliberate planning.

It is equally true that many practices have tended to drift along, motivated primarily by the general philosophy of doing what is for the good of the patient. However, a concern for financial rewards is rarely far behind, and there has always been a tendency to pursue personal goals or interests, on the ground that these are in the practice's interests.

Increasingly, business planning is undertaken by practices as the pressures on them to act as small businesses grow. This is encouraging them to make strategic decisions about how the practice should expand its activities.

The aim, quite simply, should be to shift from short-term reactive thinking, as often happens at present, to long-term and proactive planning.

WHAT IS THE PURPOSE OF PLANNING?

Planning is necessary to:

▦ achieve success; this is not something that is simply stumbled upon but is the result of active work and commitment

▦ anticipate and avoid problems; planning can identify and anticipate possible problems and help to avoid them

▦ encourage a sense of purpose; a plan encourages the practice to develop a philosophy and sense of purpose that can be understood by everyone concerned

▦ focus attention of goals; aims and targets can be defined and all members of the whole practice team can focus their efforts on achieving these

▦ build team working; planning should involve the whole practice team and is, therefore, an important tool for team building, bringing together all practice staff in shared ownership of the plan.

THE KEY QUESTIONS

When formulating a business plan, the following questions need to be addressed:

▦ Where is the practice at present, and how did it reach that position?

▦ Where does it wish to get to?

▦ How does it get there?

▦ How does it make sure it gets there?

By answering these questions, the practice can develop an overview of the tasks in hand. Turning to the immunization service, an assessment is required both of the present level of activity and of how it has evolved during recent years. However, planning cannot take place in a vacuum; there is a real market for immunization services, and their development within the practice depends on understanding this market and the role of the practice within it.

The existence of a market is obvious. Travel immunizations are offered by commercial organizations, and practices in urban areas may find that their patients use these quite extensively, especially if they are convenient for the commuter or business traveller.

Competition may also exist in child health clinic immunization services, which can put income from target payments at risk. The practice has to consider where it wants to be in the NHS market and how to achieve its objectives.

SWOT ANALYSIS[4]

This is a widely used method of analysing the current position of any business. The acronym refers to:

- Strengths

- Weaknesses

- Opportunities

- Threats.

By considering these factors, one can analyse the position of the practice. How this can be applied to an immunization service is outlined below.

Strengths

- The service is in a familiar setting that patients are used to attending for health care; practice staff are known to patients, as are the practice procedures.

---

[4]For full details of this system, see Edwards P, Jones S and Williams S (1994) *Business and Health Planning for General Practice.* Radcliffe Medical Press, Oxford.

- The service is viewed as delivering valid and trusted advice.

- There is a perceived lack of commercialization or overt financial motivation.

- Patient records are available.

- Many services can be provided free of charge to the patient.

- There is a captive market of registered patients.

Weaknesses

- There may be difficulty in arranging appointments.

- Difficulty with communication, such as telephone answering, may occur.

- Traditional surgery hours may make it difficult for those patients who work normal office hours.

- Some staff may be unsure about the importance of immunization.

- There may be poor organization within the practice.

Opportunities

- An increasing variety of vaccines is available.

- Patients have increasing travel commitments, for both business and holidays.

- There is increasing awareness of the need for immunization.

- Government campaigns heighten the uptake of immunization.

- An increasing range of travel-related opportunities to increase income is available.

Threats

- Increased competition may come from private clinics with experience in marketing.

- There is an increasing number of 'in house' clinics attached to travel agents.

- The government is considering the withdrawal of NHS provision of immunizations.

▓ Possible threats may be made to present income from item of service fees and fees from personally administered drugs.

By analysing these factors, it is possible to asses the current position and decide how it can be improved. It also enables likely future changes and the impact that these could have on the practice to be anticipated. This allows the areas that need to be tackled to be identified and prioritized.

WHERE IS THE PRACTICE HEADING?

This is where a 'mission statement' can be useful. Many GPs are cynical about the mission statements that are plastered over NHS Trust literature, most of which seem to be more like pious hopes than missions. However, mission statements can have a useful function, which are more likely to be achieved if the statements are realistic, reasonable, credible, brief and encouraging.

The very fact that such a statement needs to be produced provides a motivating factor for debate and, it is hoped, encourages the practice team as a whole to contribute to its evolution.

When writing a mission statement, several objectives have to be defined and then attained. The task of looking at how the present service falls short of the ideal enables these to be defined.

The danger is that, once the tasks that need to be done have been listed, there is an immediate temptation to rush ahead and do them all at once. This is wasteful of resources; serious consideration needs to be given to whether or not they need to be attained and, if they do, how quickly, in what order and with what consequences for other practice activities.

Objectives need to be prioritized. This task needs accurate and comprehensive information, which should be assessed objectively.

Reaching the goals

Achieving goals involves implementing the change, and successful management of this process depends on the abilities and leadership of those involved (see Table 8.1).

Table 8.1: Achieving goals

▓ Identify the services already being provided.

▓ Note any difficulties or problems.

▓ Look at strengths, weaknesses, opportunities and threats (SWOT analysis).

▓ Decide what the practice would like to attain, setting realistic targets and goals.

▓ Formulate a philosophy or a mission statement.

▓ List those changes needed to achieve this philosophy, and assess the prospects of success.

▓ Decide whether or not the resources needed to achieve these changes are available.

▓ Assess whether the change is to be radical or evolutionary.

▓ Make sure there are sufficient resources for staff training and for monitoring success.

Change can be either radical or evolutionary. An example of radical change includes a sudden decision to open a British Airways clinic in the practice or to switch to a domiciliary childhood vaccination service. Sudden changes of this kind can be threatening and desta-bilizing. Change also involves high risks, which can waste substantial resources if it fails or is poorly implemented.

The alternative is to introduce change more gradually, using a more considered approach, as summarized below.

▓ Decide what should be done, as opposed to what one would like to be done.

▓ Establish systems that can adapt to change.

▓ Monitor activity, such as immunization claims or clinic atten-dances, to identify any trends of developments that differ from expectations.

▓ Compare actual experience with projected outcomes.

▓ Set up information systems that assist future decision-making.

Making sure the practice achieves its goals

Having decided how to achieve the goals, it is important to make sure that they are actually attained. This means investing sufficient resources in the change and monitoring what is happening, so that any shortcomings can be quickly identified and corrected. Although business planning can be complex, it can be related to the development of specific services, such as the expansion of immunization services.

9

So what is marketing?

It is apparent that as general practice faces some of its biggest changes and challenges of the post-war period, the need for tighter, more professional and forward-looking management is greater than ever before. In many cases, this has meant a substantial rethink of how practices are run and how a variety of the managerial tools and techniques that previously were seen to be the prerogative of manufacturers in the private sector, and hence of little real relevance to doctors, might now possibly contribute to the better and more effective management of general practice. Prominent among these is the whole area of marketing. In many cases, however, there appears still to be a fundamental misunderstanding among doctors of precisely what marketing involves and how it might most realistically contribute either to the effective day-to-day management of the practice or, indeed, to its longer-term development.

Within this chapter, we concentrate on overcoming some of the more common preconceptions and misconceptions of marketing that we have encountered in a variety of practices and move towards developing a framework that should go some way towards establishing a stronger—and far more effective—marketing and patient-centred orientation within the practice.

Marketing is an approach to management that applies to all types of organization, since it puts the customer (in the case of general practice, of course, the patient) at the very centre of the operation and directs resources in such a way that the customer achieves a high level of satisfaction in a cost-effective manner.

When members of the public are asked to identify three or four examples of the sorts of organization that they consider to be good at marketing, the same names almost invariably crop up. Prominent among these are Coca Cola, McDonald's, Marks & Spencer and Body Shop. In the case of Coca Cola and McDonald's, both companies concentrate upon using substantial amounts of advertising to communicate clear and simple messages—'Things go better with Coke' and 'There's nothing quite like a McDonald's'—which are understood and seemingly meaningful to customers across the world. They market consistently reliable products and provide levels of service that rarely disappoint. Marks & Spencer, by contrast, has achieved a similarly strong position with little or no advertising, whilst Body Shop is successful despite spending very little on advertising, packaging or, indeed, store layout. Marketing and advertising are not, therefore, one and the same thing. Rather, advertising is just one of the marketing tools available.

On a smaller scale, think about your favourite restaurant. Although at first sight it might appear that it does not need marketing to make it successful, look more closely on your next visit at how it operates. Almost inevitably, it will have built a clear reputation as, for example, the best Italian, Indian or Chinese restaurant in town. The appearance and decor will project a clear image, the staff will be friendly, and the food and drink will have been selected to meet the demands and expectations of customers who will be made to feel comfortable in these surroundings. To create a successful restaurant, every aspect will have been planned well in advance, reflecting the owner's and manager's beliefs about what the customers they wish to attract will want. However, their task does not end there, as they will constantly be trying to improve things and make sure that every aspect of the restaurant is just right. So marketing can, but does not need to, depend on advertising and is capable of making just as important a contribution to the success of small, as well as large, organizations.

The third common misconception is that marketing is almost invariably manipulative and is selling in disguise; timeshare holiday companies are a notorious example of this. In the long term, however, customer satisfaction cannot be built on manipulation or on false promises. We may fall for it the first time but only rarely a second time. In the case of timeshare, most members of the public, and not just those who have fallen foul of the timeshare touts, are now only too aware of the typically exaggerated offers that they make and are suspicious of almost *any* offer that is made, regardless of how attractive it appears. The unfortunate result of this has, of course, been that the reputable companies in the industry (and, yes, they do exist) that offer a worthwhile product have been affected as well. Because of this, the opportunity for the market to be developed to its full potential has been lost (probably forever), not necessarily because of any failure of the product or service offered but because of the unacceptably high pressure selling techniques that have been used.

Given these examples, we should be in a far clearer position to identify what marketing in its true sense means and what it involves. Although it is difficult to list *all* of the activities that are normally covered by marketing, the most important can be identified as:

- monitoring the external environment with a view to identifying opportunities and threats

- contributing to the discussion about the nature and direction that the organization should pursue

- determining the range of products or services that should be offered

- influencing the levels of customer/patient satisfaction that are to be aimed for

- deciding upon the image that is to be projected

- managing the elements of the marketing mix on a day-to-day basis

- developing and implementing a system of feedback and control that is capable of providing a clear picture of just how well the practice is performing.

It follows from this that the essence of good marketing involves both a strong *external* and a clear *internal* orientation: external in that we are concerned with building a clear picture of what is happening, and likely to happen, outside the practice, so that we might identify and capitalize on the opportunities that exist, and internal in terms of making sure that what we offer and intend doing is feasible, and that the staff understand and are fully committed to this. Factors affecting the demand for immunization services are shown in Figure 9.1

THE TWO LEVELS OF MARKETING

If marketing is to make a significant contribution to immunization services, it needs to operate at two levels. At its most fundamental it

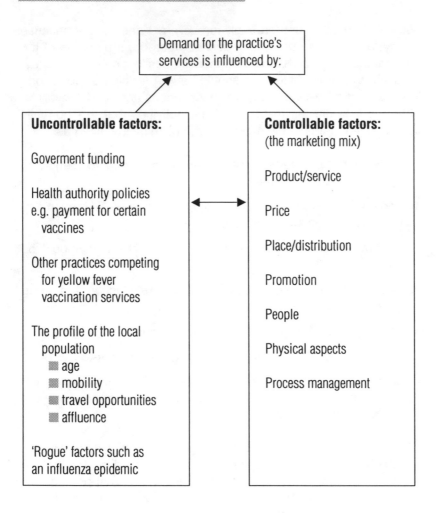

Figure 9.1: The marketing mix and the health service environment.

represents an underlying philosophy of patient satisfaction which should guide everything that doctors and staff do. On a day-to-day basis, it is concerned with issues such as the specifics of the product or service that is offered and how and where the product or service is to be presented. The essence of marketing is, therefore, to get everyone to pull together and work towards the common goal of customer/patient satisfaction. If this is done, and done effectively, the benefits can be considerable and include:

▨ higher levels of patient satisfaction

▓ a far greater likelihood of identifying market opportunities in their early stages

▓ a higher level of awareness of those factors that will ultimately prove to be a threat

▓ a better sense of direction and co-ordination

▓ a greater opportunity for staff to take more responsibility without loss of control

▓ higher levels of staff motivation as a result of their greater understanding, involvement, responsibility and commitment.

THE MARKETING PROCESS

In the light of our comments so far, we can identify the three principal strands of a marketing programme, which are:

1 the pressures of the environment (and hence the nature of any opportunities and threats that exist currently and that are likely to emerge in the future)

2 the demands, needs or expectations of patients and how these are likely to change

3 what the practice is capable of delivering.

It follows from this that the marketing process consists of four stages: analysis, planning, evaluation and implementation, and feedback and control.

Stage one: market analysis

In the first of the four stages, we need to concentrate upon developing a clear understanding of the variety of factors outside the practice. These cannot be controlled, but they determine how the practice operates and are capable of having a very real influence upon its performance; they include the general environment, the changing needs of patients and others with a say and the behaviour of competitors in the health care business. This can be summed up as 'Where are we now, and what are the demands of the environment?'

Stage two: marketing plan

Against the background of the market analysis, the emphasis needs to shift to planning and, in particular, to the identification of the goals, objectives and standards that the practice will pursue. In doing this, detailed consideration needs to be given to an assessment of the practice's capabilities, since these determine how likely it is that objectives will be met and whether any gaps exist between the practice's aspirations and objectives, and its capabilities (in other words, what one is really capable of delivering). This information can then be brought together in the form of a plan, which will be the blueprint for practice development.

Stage three: evaluation and implementation

Following this, the focus then turns to the question of how to implement the plan. It has long been recognized that the implementation stage is typically the most difficult part of the marketing planning process, since it is only too easy to lose sight of the objectives, to be blown off course by unforeseen events and to become preoccupied with day-to-day pressures, with the result that longer-term issues are ignored. A key element of marketing is, therefore, concerned with the question of how best to manage the resources that are available in as effective a manner as possible and ensure that the objectives that have been set are achieved. Because the largest and most costly resource in general practice is the staff, much of the implementation phase is, of necessity, concerned with mobilizing the staff and others, including those who supply the practice with services and products, by making sure that they understand fully what is expected of them and that they contribute fully in the most appropriate way. In other words Stage three concerns how best the objectives can be achieved and who is to be primarily responsible for them.

Stage four: feedback and control

Having implemented the marketing plan, attention then needs to be paid to measuring the performance levels that have been achieved, with a view to identifying any need for modification and improvement. There is, therefore, a need to monitor performance under a variety of headings. These might include:

■ financial performance of immunization services, including income, expenditure and profitability

■ doctors' commitments and performance

■ staff performance, including turnover, attitudes, motivation, development and training

■ patient management, including the demand for services

■ premises management, including their suitability and the nature of any improvements made

■ the development of new services

■ the introduction of new or modified patient management systems.

In summary, what check and balances can be put into the system to ensure that it is known how well the plan is operating?

DEVELOPING THE PATIENT-CENTRED PRACTICE: THE FIRST FEW STEPS

In order to develop a marketing-oriented and truly patient-centred practice, there is an obvious need to understand in detail the market for primary health care and, in particular, the sorts of factors that are likely to lead to higher levels of patient satisfaction. Without this information, any marketing effort will be unfocused and, at best, of only limited value. So what is it that contributes to patient satisfaction? Although most doctors would argue that they have a clear idea of this, it is only the patients themselves who are *really* able to answer the question. Lessons can be learned from the commercial sector that provide some help in going about this.

When dealing with a commercial client, one can begin by posing a deceptively simple question: what *benefits* are the customers really looking for? The significance of this is that rarely, if ever, do people buy a product or service for its own sake. Instead, they buy it for the benefits that it provides. Perhaps the most commonly cited example of this is the purchase of a drill, which, as the American management guru Theodore Levitt pointed out in the 1950s, is bought not for its physical qualities but in order to provide holes.

By the same token, cars such as Porsche, Mercedes, BMW and Jaguar, whether we like to admit it or not, are bought as much for their status, image and prestige as for anything else; customers then justify their purchase by highlighting features such as the build quality, the pre- and post-sales services, reliability and so on. Equally, research in the expensive, boxed chocolate market reveals that buying motives are seldom concerned with taste but are more commonly to do with the perceived value of the product as a gift. In the case of the beer market, the primary buying motives among 18–22-year-olds have consistently been shown to be concerned not with the beer's taste or strength but with the images associated with the brand and peer group pressure.

Recognition of this highlights the need for a clear and detailed understanding of the distinctions that exist between features and benefits, since it is this understanding that underpins any attempt to develop a truly patient-centred practice. It is, for example, only too easy to talk about the sort of thing that GPs do (the features) rather than what patients get from it (the benefits). This is likely to be manifested in terms of how a doctor cures an illness—the cure being the *feature*. However, looking at it from the patients' point of view, they go to a GP feeling unwell. The only reason that they will consider immunization is for the perceived benefits that it offers, so their perception of such benefits is fundamental.

Coming to terms with the benefits

In thinking about the nature and significance of benefits, Herzberg's two-factor theory of motivation can be of some help. The theory distinguishes between *satisfiers* (factors that create satisfaction) and *dissatisfiers* (factors that create dissatisfaction). In the case of a car, for example, the absence of a warranty would be a dissatisfier. The existence of a warranty, however, is not a satisfier, since it is not one of the principal reasons for buying the product. Instead, as we suggested earlier, these are more likely to be the car's looks, its performance and the status that the driver feels it lends.

There are several implications of this theory for the marketing of general practice, the two most significant of which are, first, that the seller (that is, the doctor and the practice) needs to be fully aware of the dissatisfiers which, while they will not by themselves sell the product, can easily 'unsell' it. The second implication, which follows logically from this, is that the doctor and the practice staff need to understand in detail the various satisfiers and then concentrate not just upon supplying them, but also giving emphasis to them so that patients are fully aware of them.

It should be apparent from this that achieving a truly patient-centred immunization service is a potentially difficult task, and for most practices, is likely to involve significant changes in operating practices and culture. However, aspects of such a practice are shown in the list on page 93.

■ What are the principal satisfiers and dissatisfiers within the practice?

■ What are we doing/can we do to increase the satisfiers and reduce or abolish completely the dissatisfiers?

■ What are the obstacles to making the sorts of changes needed in order to achieve a patient-centred practice, how significant are they, and how might we overcome them?

There are several issues that emerge from these findings, the three most significant of which are that a remarkably high proportion of patients believe that doctors do not really listen enough, do not explain things fully and do not spend sufficient time on the consultation. A comparison across Europe of how much consultation time is spent with the patient paints an interesting picture: in France doctors spend an average of 20 minutes with each patient, in Germany 18 minutes, in Italy 12, and in the UK just 6. Although the obvious reaction to this, and indeed the one that is encountered on numerous occasions in our work with GPs, is that the time is simply not there, this response misses the significance of the point being raised and, of course, runs counter to the idea of the patient-centred practice.

Moving ahead

Given the nature of these comments, the question of how the truly patient-centred practice might be developed needs to be approached by considering the answers to a series of questions.

▓ Do we *really* know what levels of satisfaction and dissatisfaction currently exist among our patients?

▓ Where patients are dissatisfied, do we *really* know how deep and/or justified this dissatisfaction is?

▓ Are we *really* aware of the causes of patient irritation with the practice, and are there any common strands between any causes for complaint/dissatisfaction that patients might have?

▓ Do we *really* understand what leads to high(er) levels of patient satisfaction?

▓ Would we *really* be willing to make possible radical changes in how we operate in order to achieve higher levels of patient satisfaction?

▓ Have we *really* done enough to train our staff, or do we rely upon common sense and learning from the long-established members of the practice?

▓ How much money would we *really* be willing to invest in training and facilities in order to achieve higher levels of patient satisfaction?

The answers to the questions posed in this chapter, will lead to some understanding of the nature of the practice's orientation and the extent to which it really is patient-centred. Experience has shown that practices can be viewed very broadly in terms of a continuum, ranging from the inward looking, old-fashioned practice, in which patients know their place and dare not move from at one end, through to the highly patient-centred practice at the other.

The **doctor-centred** pratice is characterized by a belief that:

- general practice has not really changed since the 1930s and change is something that should be resisted

- patients are fundamentally a nuisance

- surgery hours should be based on what is most convenient to the partners

- the practice manager and reception staff are there to keep patients away from the doctors as much as possible

- the surgery building is regarded as a cost, which must be kept to a minimum, rather than an investment

- doctors always know best.

The **patient-centred** service is characterized by:

- a clear understanding of how the patients' full range of needs might best be satisfied and of the benefits they are seeking

- a willingness to adapt the practice and its operating approaches to meet these needs fully

- an understanding of how rival practices operate and what can be learned from them

- a willingness to experiment

- a listening approach

- the development of new and patient-relevant services

- an appointments system that is designed to suit patients' needs

- a willingness to invest in better facilities, including the waiting room

- a well thought out programme of training for medical and non-medical staff.

10

Auditing the service

The two key resources that are constantly being juggled within general practice are time and money.

There is no doubt that recent NHS changes have made the profession far more financially aware, and the perception of general practice as a small business has spread rapidly. If a practice is to run efficiently, one aim should be to ensure that income is maximized and expenditure minimized; in short, the business is run as profitably as possible. Naturally, this objective must be balanced against the profession's ethical obligation to practise good medicine. This view of general practice is unexceptional and does not differ from the philosophy of any small business. However, unlike in other commercial enterprises, in medicine the care and treatment of the patient must take priority over financial factors.

GPs' growing awareness of financial matters has been accompanied by a realization that time is an even more finite resource. To individual GPs, 'time' appears to be an inelastic commodity, as more and more demands are made upon them. First, there are growing demands on their clinical time, because patients expect greater access to their doctors and ask for new treatments and investigations. Consultation rates are increasing, and new screening programmes and health promotion schemes are being introduced.

There is also an increasing demand on GPs' time for management purposes. Fund holding greatly increases the time spent on administrative tasks and registration, and all practices are having to spend more time on management tasks, negotiations, clinical review and analysis and health care planning. Add to all this the ever more onerous out-of-hours commitment demanded, and the increased pressures of family life, and the stereotype of the GP on the golf course is fast becoming a sick joke!

Because time and money are valuable resources, it is important to ensure that they are not squandered. Any steps that enable a practice to ensure it is using these scarce commodities as effectively as possible must be welcomed. This is why the process of audit is so important, because it provides precisely the information that is required to assess whether or not a practice is being managed effectively.

It is unfortunate that the term 'audit' carries regulatory and managerial overtones and that this impression has been reinforced by the fact that audit is used by NHS management to monitor and control the service. This should not alter the fact that it is a powerful and valuable management tool, which, if correctly used, can produce enormous benefits for the practice and the individual GP.

The benefits of audit include:

▧ assessing how effectively the practice is currently being run

▧ analysing the cost–benefit ratio of a decision to invest time or money in a particular activity

▧ clarifying internal processes and procedures

▧ identifying gaps in the services provided

▧ identifying any opportunities to earn income that are currently being missed.

If it is accepted as a valuable tool, audit can be applied to a wide range of activities, including immunization.

Planning audit

If audit is undertaken in isolation for its own sake, it is unrewarding, frustrating and inaccurate, because those involved lack motivation. This means that before even considering undertaking an audit, there must be interest in and commitment to the process.

Defining what is to be audited

GPs should look at an activity that is a matter of repeated concern and of interest to the whole practice. If they intend to encourage their staff to become involved in audit, it is useful to choose a topic that is relevant to their work, for example the appointment system. The simpler the audit being undertaken, the easier and more rewarding the process. Often it is issues of immediate concern, or areas in which problems continually occur, that are most likely to benefit from the audit process.

Deciding who will undertake the audit

There is no reason why audit should not be undertaken by any member of the practice team. As long as he or she knows what procedures need to be followed and is sufficiently motivated, anyone can be encouraged to do it.

Deciding on how the audit is to be done

The way in which information is collected, and by whom, determines who is going to do most of the spade work. The need for reliable information means that data collection should be done by those who are most interested and motivated to do it.

Planning for the results

There is little point in carrying out an audit merely for the sake of gathering information. The whole essence of audit is that it should identify weaknesses that need to be addressed and act as a catalyst for change. The need for change may become apparent as the audit progresses, and it is important to accept that the final results may challenge well-established working practices and lead to change. If this premise is not accepted at the outset, the whole process becomes pointless.

THE AUDIT PROCESS

Defining the aims and standards a practice aspires to reach

A practice may, for example, aim to ensure that all adults have had a primary course of tetanus and polio immunization.

Looking at those elements of performance that need to be measured

In this example, the practice would need to measure the proportion of patients whose notes record that a primary course of immunization has been given.

Considering whether there is a need for change

What should be done to enable the aim to be met? Adult patients need to be asked specifically about their vaccination status, and there needs to be an increased awareness of the need to provide immunization services to a category of patients who were previously neglected, for this purpose.

Determining the required resources

These may be financial or time resources. Often the most important resource is the commitment and enthusiasm of the staff member who is implementing the change by drawing up a plan to call up those who need immunization or a protocol for the practice to implement. Alternatively, it could be a financial resource, such as the provision of a refrigerator in each consulting room, to encourage opportunistic vaccination.

Assessing achieved improvement in performance

This can be assessed by examining the proportion of patients who now satisfy the original objective after the change has been implemented. This will enable the practice to assess the effectiveness of its improved procedures.

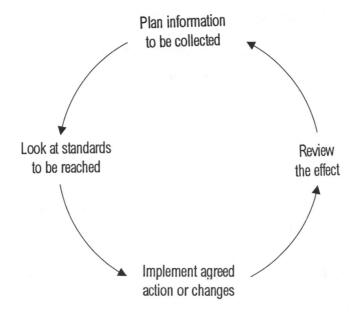

Figure 10.1: The audit process.

The audit process works like a loop (Figure 10.1). Once the area to be audited has been defined, information should be gathered to assess what is currently going on. However, just collecting information, calculating results and reaching conclusions is not the end of the matter. The essential task is to use the results to initiate change and, equally importantly, to repeat the audit some time later to see whether or not the change has had the desired effect.

Audit is not a static isolated procedure; it is a powerful tool that should be applied repeatedly to monitor and improve performance. A simple and easy way of thinking about how continuous audit might work is to consider computerized audit.

Take, for example, the case of childhood immunization. Information about the levels of immunization reached is important both clinically, through protecting children against infectious disease, and financially, with respect to the target payments that are a significant proportion of many practices' income. There are also important matters concerning the effectiveness of the practice's policies for recalling patients and chasing defaulters. The entire audit process can be computerized if the child immunization records are themselves computerized. The advantages of computerized audit is that once it is set up, the audit cycle can be regularly repeated whenever the practice wants.

A computerized audit cycle works as follows:

- enter the audit on the computer and run the procedure

- study the results, noting the levels reached

- consider whether or not there is a need for telephone recalls or any other steps to persuade defaulters to attend, and implement whatever action is required

- repeat the audit, to see whether targets are now being reached.

The last two can be repeated until either targets are met or it is decided that the effort required to achieve them is not justified by the potential clinical or financial gain.

Even without the benefits of computers, repeated audits can be undertaken; for example, a questionnaire can be used to monitor the convenience of travel clinic appointment times, and any necessary changes can be introduced. By repeating the survey and looking at patient satisfaction levels, a practice can see whether or not the available appointment times are more appropriate.

TYPES OF AUDIT

There are three aspects of any activity that need to be audited; these are:

- structure

- process

- outcome.

Structure

This refers to the actual bricks, mortar, rooms and facilities. With respect to immunization services, all of these may need to be audited. For example, by reviewing the facilities available for the child immunization clinic, it is possible to identify any shortcomings that may discourage parents from attending, such as difficulty of access, a lack of a ramp or buggy park, a lack of toys or seats for children and an unwelcoming atmosphere.

Process

This aspect concerns the actual services and includes virtually everything that goes on within the surgery. Not only is each task in itself a process that can be identified for the purposes of the audit, but also each main task can be subdivided into smaller tasks. For example, it may be decided to audit the use of form FP73. This would involve the following process.

■ Form FP73 is completed by computer or by staff.

■ FP73 is signed by the GP.

■ The completed form is sent to the health authority or a health board for reimbursement.

Each of these stages can be regarded as having its own subtasks, which can also be audited.

■ Who fills in form FP73?

■ Are the patient details accurate and legible?

■ How accurate is the country of destination?

■ Are the vaccine batch numbers correct?

■ Are all the forms signed by the correct doctor?

■ Are all the forms dated?

Process auditing is particularly useful for looking at the efficiency and completeness of a practice's administrative systems.

Outcome

In most areas of medicine outcomes are difficult to define precisely and there is often disagreement about how to measure success or failure. How does a doctor audit the success of a migraine clinic—by a reduced number of attacks, by reduced severity of attacks, by the number of days off work or by reduced drug consumption? There are arguments for and against all of these criteria.

Immunization is an area that has the advantage of a comparatively accurate and objective end point, namely the administration of the vaccine to the patient: a patient has either had a tetanus immunization or he or she has not, has received an influenza vaccine or has not. As such, there are fairly precise outcome measures, which make audit in this area comparatively easy. However, there are some exceptions; for example, rubella and hepatitis B immunizations may only be regarded as having been successful on evidence of seroconversion.

HOW TO AUDIT IMMUNIZATION SERVICES

The importance of auditing immunization services can be illustrated by some examples of how audit can improve their quality or profitability.

Financial audits

Staffing a clinic

Aim: to determine whether extra staff would boost clinic income.

Performance: calculate the cost of increasing the staff budget. Determine what direct reimbursement, if any, can be expected, and what the cost of an extra member of staff would be, including salary, tax, national insurance and other overheads. Calculate benefits likely to accrue from the tasks that will be performed, for example, more patients are seen and more immunizations are given, there is increased selling of travel packs to private patients or better advice and more thorough protection can be given.

Changes: weigh the cost against the clinical and financial benefits, in both the short and the long term. Look at the development of the service.

Resources: are the resources available to support an increase in cost?

Review performance: are the costs now justified by the increasing income or better quality of work-load? If not, can the change be reversed?

Reimbursement for vaccination

Aim: to make sure that prescriptions are written for reimbursement of those vaccines that are personally administered and to avoid any financial loss to the practice.

Performance: record all immunizations that are given, by a computerized search of immunization records, over a period of one month. Do this for either all vaccines or one specific vaccine (in which case an expensive vaccine should be chosen, such as active hepatitis A, for which the greatest losses might be occurring). Having worked out how many doses of the vaccine(s) have been given, this figure should be compared with the number of doses submitted to the Prescription Pricing Authority for reimbursement at the end of the month.

Change: review the results, and consider what measures are needed to ensure that prescriptions are written.

Resources: should there be more time for each appointment, better staff training, allocation of the responsibility to a different member of staff?

Review performance: repeat the audit to check whether or not there has been an improvement and that a prescription is now written for each immunization. This audit will need to be repeated frequently to ensure that the system does not lead to financial losses caused by forgotten prescriptions.

Clinical audit

Influenza immunization

Aim: all those who are at risk of influenza to be immunized annually.

Performance: use the disease register or computer to find all those patients who conform to the recommended criteria for influenza immunization. Compare these with the numbers that have actually received the immunization and produce a list of those who would benefit from being offered the vaccine.

Change: more effective calling up of patients or introduction of different clinics at more suitable times.

Resources: are rooms and staff available? Is the cost of postage or telephone calls justified?

Review performance: review one month later and see what proportion of patients has still not been offered protection. In addition, compare new systems year by year.

Administrative audit

Clinic satisfaction

Aim: to ensure that patients are able to make an appointment to receive their immunizations within a short time or at a convenient time, and that they can get an appointment within 24 hours or an appointment within three working days.

Performance: carry out a daily check of available appointments in the immunization clinic for that day. Check evening or early morning appointments for the next three days. Question patients as they come for their appointment regarding their satisfaction.

Change: adjust the number of available appointment or hours of the clinic to more accurately reflect demand. Change the times of the clinic or open at weekends.

Resources: overtime from staffing the surgery late in the evening. Security precautions, heat and light.

Review performance: look at level of service usage. Question patients about service and see whether or not alterations have resulted in benefit to the practice or patients.

Index